Insomnia

Author

CONTENTS

Introduction   4

Normal Sleep   7

The Effects of Too Little Sleep   16

Why Don't You Go to Sleep?   19

Self-help for Insomnia   26

How to Control your Mind and Relax   35

Pills, Medicines and Sleep   42

Some Odd Aids to Sleep   57

How to Deal with your Insomnia   62

    STAGE 1 - Are you a true or a false insomniac?   62

    STAGE 2 - Why are you not sleeping?   64

    STAGE 3 - Take away the cause of your insomnia   66

    STAGE 4 - Is your insomnia acute or chronic?   68

    STAGE 5a - Treatment for acute insomnia   69

    STAGE 5b - Treatment of chronic insomnia   71

    STAGE 6 - Making the most of your insomnia   74

Introduction

Do you suffer from insomnia? Half the population do at some time in their lives, and at any one time one in six have problems in sleeping. Even those who do not normally have any difficulty in getting to sleep have times when they lie awake much longer than they would like, often before a big occasion when they want to be at their best. So you can hardly say the subject does not concern you. If we could abolish difficulty in sleeping from our lives we would all feel more secure.

By definition insomnia is habitual sleeplessness, difficulty in sleeping that goes on night after night and often seems to have no end. But this usually starts gradually; you take an hour to get off to sleep instead of your more usual half-hour, you wake up in the night but do not drop off to sleep again immediately, you notice that with less sleep you cannot concentrate and are not as efficient the next day. There may be a perfectly good reason why you start off having difficulty in sleeping but once the pattern of insomnia has been established it tends to repeat itself. The critical time comes when you begin to worry about not sleeping. Then it feeds on itself. Worry makes insomnia worse, which leads to more worry, and so the vicious cycle goes on. To cure insomnia you have to break this cycle and the earlier it is done the better.

There are many ways of tackling insomnia, and it is likely that one or more of them will be relevant to you. But to solve any problem you have to be aware of its nature. If your car breaks down you need to know something about its normal working if you are going to fix what is wrong. The insomniac has to do much more than read down a list of remedies and try each of them at random.

Understanding insomnia involves many steps. First you need to know about normal sleep, what happens when you suffer from sleep loss, and the many different causes of insomnia. Then you can move on to choosing a treatment for your particular problem instead of picking one out of the blue. In the course of this investigation, and it is just as much an investigation as solving a mathematical problem, you may find there is a great deal more to your insomnia than just difficulty in sleeping. It can be tied up with your sex life, your work, or your whole life-style.

The complaint of insomnia is, then, just the tip of the iceberg. Below the surface there is a mass of other problems which will need sorting out before you can sleep soundly again. On the other hand your insomnia may have a trivial cause. Perhaps your bedroom is too cold, your bed is the wrong one for you, or you sleep with someone who snores. The reason for not sleeping may be quite obvious or completely obscure, but do not be afraid to look at all the possibilities first before deciding what to do.

Many years ago it was thought that a fever, or high temperature, was a disease. Treatment was concentrated on trying to bring the high temperature down. If someone died in this state, the fever was said to be the cause. With greater medical knowledge, we now know literally hundreds of causes of fever and bringing the temperature down by ice packs, sponging with cold water or similar methods is a minor part of treatment. The important thing is to find the medical disease causing the fever and then give the treatment for that disease. If you look at insomnia in the same sort of way you will realize that a lot of questions have to be asked first before treatment is given. In many ways the word 'treatment' is unfortunate, because it implies that there is some special cure for the problem, to be given by an expert with superior knowledge. In fact, in most cases of insomnia you will be asking all the questions and providing all the answers. There is no need for outside help, you have the means of solving the problem at your disposal. You will get nowhere if you look at insomnia as a province for the medical, or any other, profession, presenting it to them like a crossword puzzle waiting to be completed. Whatever help is given by others, you are going to have to take the lion's share. After all, it is your sleep that is at stake.

There will be some who read this book who will realize that they are not true insomniacs after all. Although they complain of delay in getting to sleep, they do not suffer any of the problems of sleep loss during the day. This may be because they expect more sleep than necessary. There is great variation in the amount of sleep each of us needs and many of us could function quite well on less than we are getting at present. If you expect eight hours' sleep and only need six you should not be surprised if you have some problems in getting to sleep. These people have the easiest solution of all; they just need to go to bed a little later than usual.

There are some others who will be more reluctant to admit they are phony insomniacs. These are people who insist that they spend hours lying awake at night, often never sleeping a wink, yet they have a full night's sleep. This can be proved by special tests involving the recording of brain waves. Brain waves can tell us when someone is asleep or not and we shall come across them again later. Recordings of brain waves can be taken for a whole night and the amount of sleep totted up over this period. It is a much more reliable way of telling how much sleep you have had than your own ideas on the subject. You might find it hard to believe that your memory has let you down. Some people claim that they must have been awake all night because they heard a clock chime on the hour for each hour of the night. The sleep tests show that they did indeed wake eight times at hourly intervals and were awake for five minutes following each chiming. But for the remaining fifty-five minutes in each hour they were fast asleep. Therefore instead of having eight hours' sleep they only had seven hours and twenty minutes' sleep, but this can hardly be called insomnia. The reason our memories let us down is because we cannot remember anything when we are asleep (apart from dreams, and then only in part). That is why people who are very sleepy say things like, 'I just laid my head on the pillow and the next thing

I knew it was morning.' So before you consider yourself a real insomniac make certain you are not in the phony group. If you sleep with someone else they can often tell you for how long you sleep each night, although unless they stay awake all night they cannot give you a complete record. But they can often have a good idea when you first drop off to sleep. If you think it takes you two hours to get off to sleep and your partner's independent evidence suggests it is only twenty minutes, their measurement is probably the more accurate.

Even if you do not have insomnia you are likely to know someone well who does. True insomnia causes a great deal of suffering, suffering which is often forgotten, ignored or even made fun of by others. After reading this book you may have a better idea of the extent of this distress, and may be able to offer a few words of advice.

If you feel each night when you go to bed that you are about to enter a dark, silent world about which nothing is known, then you are bound to be unsettled or even a little frightened, and this does no good for insomnia.

Of course, as most chronic insomniacs already know, having an encyclopedic knowledge about sleep and sleep disorders is not going to solve the problems of sleeplessness.

By thinking of all the different ways of getting off to sleep you are actually keeping yourself awake, as your mind is being kept active. Like turning off all the lights before going to bed at night, sleep is a closing down process. You want to draw the curtains across your mind and let it go to sleep, but every time you think about it you are opening the curtains again! The trick of 'switching off' your mind is one which Western society has completely failed to master. All the apparent success of our society is based on activity, power, industry, technology and other positive things which involve the mind working hard, if not on overload. If some of us find it difficult to turn down the power when needed, our Western philosophy cannot provide an answer. But for centuries the countries of the East have been developing and perfecting the techniques of 'switching off, which are now part of their religious and cultural life. Rather too late we have discovered the advantages of these techniques, and expect to have them taught to us immediately by our local 'guru'!

Unfortunately they are not so easy to learn by Westerners of a completely different life-style, and even those who opt out entirely from our thrusting, aggressive society find it difficult to adjust to a new one in the East. Still, there are many treatments for insomnia which have developed from the religious and philosophical concepts of Buddhism, Shintoism and Hinduism and these are described in a later chapter.

Above all I would like to think that reading this book will give you a balanced picture of insomnia, neither exaggerating nor minimizing its causes, effects or difficulties.

We have to remember that we are dealing with a manmade problem; as far as we know insomnia is not suffered to any degree by other animals. Sleep is a natural state for every living organism-something very like it occurs in plants as well-and without it we should all become exhausted and pack up altogether. In treating insomnia we are only trying to add a little extra sleeping time to the hours of sleep enjoyed by all people, and that includes insomniacs as well, so that they are better able to live their lives. Once the insomniac has been shoved out of his sleepless groove the natural processes of sleep should take over again and maintain the balance between rest and activity. As long as you remember that getting out of the groove involves your efforts at least as much as those of others, eventually you should be successful. Sound sleep is a right, not a luxury.

Normal Sleep

It used to be thought that sleep was a simple state of affairs. Because little can be remembered during sleep it was natural to think that all the systems in the body slowed down to base-line levels and stayed like this till you woke up in the morning.

Now we realize that sleep is complicated and a great deal has to go on in mind and body if it is to do its job effectively.

First let us go through a typical eight-hour sleep as experienced by a good sleeper. When he gets into bed he probably feels tired and is usually relaxed. He turns the light off and takes up his favorite sleeping position.

There are lots of different sleeping positions and there is little to choose between them. One of the commonest is to curl up with your hands between your knees and your head bent forwards. It has been pointed out that this position is the same as that taken up by babies before birth in their mothers' wombs, and various theories have suggested that going to sleep is like going back into the womb.

Of course there may be a more obvious explanation. You get warmer more quickly in a bunched-up position and warmth is necessary for good sleep. Other positions include lying flat on your back with your legs stretched out like a mummy, on your side with your hands together underneath your face (this makes children look very innocent and appealing and is much loved by parents), and complicated positions with arms and legs all over the place. Some people get warm very quickly in bed and search out the cool parts with their bodies until they often take up the whole bed, even if it is a double one. You will know what I mean if you have to share a bed with someone like this. Once you have found the right sleeping position, and many take several minutes to find the ideal one, the eyes are closed and within a few minutes you start to doze.

During dozing your mind wanders from subject to subject and you never hold any train of thought for long. While you are dozing you often drift in and out of sleep without realizing it. The actual dividing line between being asleep and awake is not clear cut and it is impossible to tell when it has taken place. At this stage the slightest stimulus, like a light touch, a draught blowing on the cheek or a creak in the door can bring you back to full waking. This can even happen when you have been asleep for a few minutes and on waking you would probably insist that you had been awake all the time. This is yet another piece of evidence that your memory is not to be trusted when you are in bed sleeping, or trying to get to sleep, and insomniacs should take note.

In the first stage of sleep proper (which in most people is reached within thirty minutes after going to bed) you are relaxed, your heart is beating slowly and you are unaware of things around you. You may move around in the bed and change your sleeping position but your movements tend to be slow. But it only needs a slight stimulus, such as a clock chiming or a heavy lorry passing in the road outside, to wake you up again. It is not just the amount of stimulus that matters, it is novelty that counts. If a stimulus stands out from the background it is much more likely to wake you.

About an hour after you have gone to sleep you reach the deepest stage, when you are completely relaxed, your heart is beating more slowly still, your breathing is slow and completely regular, and you no longer move during your sleep. This is the stage at which the sleeper is said to be 'dead to the world'. It is extremely difficult to wake stimulation. If you are forced into waking at this stage, such as, for example, by a telephone ringing by your bed, you will take some time to become fully awake.

You may reply to the telephone call before you are fully aware of what you are saying, and give an answer which can be complete nonsense or at least quite different from the reply you would have made in full consciousness.

Once you have reached this deepest stage of sleep you might expect to stay in this stage until morning. But this is not what happens, and for the remaining hours of your sleep an extraordinary sequence of events occurs. This was first found out by research workers in America with the aid of recordings of brain waves, and it is worth telling in some detail. As we mentioned earlier, the brain waves can tell whether we are asleep or not. More than this, they tell us which stage of sleep we are in. They are recorded by sticking silver discs on the scalp and measuring the electrical changes going on in the brain. When we are awake the brain waves are very fast, but the sleepier we get the slower they become. When you are in the deepest stages of sleep the brain waves are at their slowest and most regular. A glance at the brain waves can tell us which stage of sleep someone is in and is more reliable than just looking at someone while they are asleep.

Now the research workers in America found when they recorded the brain waves of people for the whole of a normal night's sleep that some very peculiar things happened. First of all, as we have already described, you fall asleep after about twenty minutes and as your sleep gets deeper your brain waves get slower. At this stage the researchers sat back and prepared to see the same slow pattern of brain waves continue until morning. They were quite surprised to see something different. Instead of staying slow and regular the brain waves start to speed up again. They continue in this way until, about thirty minutes after the deepest stage of sleep, or ninety minutes after first going off to sleep, the brain waves are the same as in the first sleep stage. As sleep becomes lighter you start breathing more rapidly, your heart rate increases and you start changing your position in bed again. Then, even more surprisingly, you go through a phase in which you act as though you are awake, but are, in fact, still asleep.

No, it is not sleep-walking; we shall come across that later. During this phase you will probably open your eyes and look from side to side as if seeing something. You are restless and may even thrash about the bed, your heart rate and breathing increase to that of your normal waking state. This stage of sleep is commonly called REM sleep

(REM stands for rapid eye movements, which are the most distinctive features of this stage of sleep).

You often become sexually excited during REM sleep and in men the penis becomes erect. Dreaming takes place mainly during REM sleep but although sexual interest is aroused at the same time you should not assume that all dreams are sexual ones. Oddly enough, although REM sleep appears to be light sleep it is more difficult to wake someone up at this time. If you are woken you can often recall your dreams in graphic detail. This period lasts for about fifteen minutes. After this the whole cycle repeats itself for the rest of the night. So during the course of our normal eight hours of sleep there are about four cycles, each with its phases of deep sleep, light sleep and REM sleep. In sleep, as in life, nothing is ever still for long. In most of us the deepest stages of sleep are reached and last longer in the first two cycles, following which the proportion of time spent in the deep stages gets less. In the four hours before we wake up deep sleep may not occur at all.

What is the purpose of our peculiar rhythm of sleep? Does it give us any advantages or is it just a meaningless merry-go-round? Some hints about its development have come from watching sleeping babies. Sleeping and waking in babies also follows a similar cycle, except that in each period of ninety minutes just under half the time is spent awake.

This cycle lasts throughout the twenty-four-hour day. What occurs in adults appears to be the same basic cycle, but as it would be too disrupting to wake up every hour -and a half, sleep continues even during the times that the brain seems to be in a waking state. It is not certain whether the need to dream is an important part of sleep, and the significance of dreaming in general has caused a lot of argument. Dreams are part of our normal sleep and we all dream for about two hours each night, although much of our dreaming is not recalled. Some people are certain that they do not dream at all. If you feel this way try keeping a pencil and paper by your bedside at night and writing down your impressions immediately- and I stress immediately- you wake up in the morning or at times during the night. You will be surprised how many dreams you can recall. Most dreams consist of a distorted memory of events of the previous waking day mixed with apparently fictitious material which we realize is false when we wake up but which we think has real substance while we are asleep. Some people have even put forward the view that our dreams are our real life and what happens during the day is only a dream!

Nightmares or unpleasant dreams are more likely to occur if we are brooding about nasty things during the previous day or when going off to sleep. Similarly, we are more likely to have pleasant dreams if the previous day's experiences have been happy ones. All dreams involve visual images, many involve hearing as well; some people always dream in color, others only in black and white. As a black-and-white dreamer I have always been envious of those who dream in color. Even the blind can dream in color so it is an ability that depends on visual imagination rather than vision itself.

Some psychiatrists and psychologists feel that the contents of dreams are important because they tell us what is going on in our unconscious mind. According to theories first put forward by Sigmund Freud the conscious mind suppresses threatening and unacceptable thoughts, wishes and impulses during our waking life and dumps them in the dustbin of the unconscious. When we are asleep the suppression is less effective, off comes the lid of the dustbin and the unconscious can express itself in dreams. When we wake up the conscious mind immediately takes over again and our recall of the dream becomes distorted because the suppressors have started working again. Nevertheless, enough can be reconstructed by analysing the dream as we recall it to expose the underlying ferment and torment in the unconscious mind.

Freud called the analysis of dreams 'the royal road to the unconscious' as no other approach lets us get so close to the innermost secrets of the mind.

Others hold a completely different view that dreams have no meaning in themselves and merely represent the brain 'running over' the events of the previous day in an accelerated and random fashion. What we remember when we wake is an attempt to make sense of rubbish, of information which is a hotchpotch of memories of recent and distant events, feelings and attitudes. It is as though a vacuum cleaner was going through the cupboards of your mind, sucking up a lot of bits and pieces you hardly knew were there, and generally stirring up dust in the process of cleaning. A similar process of 'spring-cleaning' goes on in large computers when they are having their memory banks cleared, and the information produced contains about the same amount of part sense, part nonsense, that occurs in dreams.

Sleep-talking and sleep-walking are other things which are also often linked with dreams. Sleep-talking usually happens during REM sleep and often the words spoken can be linked with the dream you are having. If you are woken up at the time you are sleep-talking the dream which is recalled is seen to fit into the sequence. Similarly, sleepwalking is often considered to be the acting out of a dream.

The clearest example of this that I have come across was a person who jumped straight through a closed first-floor bedroom window in the middle of the night for no apparent reason. He was thought at first to have attempted suicide but then he explained that he was having a dream about being caught in a fire. In his dream he was trapped by fire and the only way he could escape was by jumping out of the window. He woke up just as he went through the glass and crashed to the concrete outside, breaking a leg and several ribs. There have even been some cases in which murders have been said to have been committed while under the influence of sleep-walking. In these rare cases the apparent murderer could not be convicted as he was not conscious of what he was doing at the time of the offence. Sleep-walking also happens in deeper stages of sleep, often going on for many months without the sleepwalker or others knowing about it. Do not be too concerned if you sleep-walk, for in itself it does not mean you have any mental or physical disturbance. It is common among young children and tends to get less as you grow older.

Various body functions alter with each stage of sleep. We have already mentioned that your heart rate slows in the deepest stages; in REM sleep the rate increases and is sometimes quite fast during an emotional dream. The sexual excitement during REM sleep may lead to a 'wet dream' in men and masturbation in women. In a wet dream the penis becomes erect, followed by thrusting movements ending with the ejaculation of semen. Women also have erotic dreams but with less dramatic consequences.

You may be having an openly sexual dream at the time often accompanied by a fantasy of the sexual act.

Frequently the dream is not erotic or you cannot re member it. There is often a great deal of guilt after the wet dream has been discovered, particularly in teenagers who are just getting used to an increase in sexual feelings. In fact you should not feel guilty but be reassured that you are sexually normal. It is interesting that fully grown men who complain of impotence may have wet dreams while they are asleep, which emphasizes that there is nothing wrong with their sexual organs. Their psychological inhibitions prevent normal sex when awake but are suppressed during sleep.

During deep sleep your breathing slows down considerably. The rate of breathing is, to a large extent, determined by the amount of carbon dioxide in the body, the waste gas that leaves the body by passing through the blood into the lungs and is then breathed out. As carbon dioxide itself in large amounts makes us sleepy, some people think that in order to become sleepy we need to have excess carbon dioxide in our bodies. Although this is generally untrue-most athletes do not drop off to sleep during training-there are a few unusual people who sleep excessively and who have too much carbon dioxide in their bodies even during waking life. The condition is sometimes called the Pickwickian syndrome, after the fat boy, Joe, in *Pickwick Papers,* who, from Dickens' description, is a prime example. Joe, you may remember, was fat, red-faced and permanently drowsy. He spent most of his time asleep, and when not asleep he was usually eating.

The only stimulus that aroused him to wakefulness spontaneously was the smell of food and if no meal was likely he would rapidly return to slumber. Even while eating appetizing helpings of veal, ham or pigeon-pie he could still fall asleep only to start chewing again on waking. It is thought that the excessive weight of these sleepy, fat people leads to inefficient breathing so that carbon dioxide tends to build up, but it should be remembered that fat people tend to be more settled and sleepy individuals than those who are thin even if their breathing is quite normal.(This is not an invitation to insomniacs to grow fat and sleep well, as the relationship does not always work.) In a chapter concerned with normal sleeping it would be wrong not to mention snoring, which many people have to suffer. As snoring only happens during sleep the snorer never complains, and may even deny that he (or she) snores. But to the insomniac who shares the bed (or house for those sonorous snoozers whose snores reverberate from room to room) it is a continuous reminder that someone is blissfully asleep while they lie awake in frustration.

It is like Tantalus of Greek legend, condemned to remain hungry and thirsty in Hades with food and water just out of his reach. In the same way, the insomniac lying next to the snorer is just as close and yet so far from sleep. One woman I know insisted her insomnia would be cured if she only had the courage to give physical expression to these pent-up feelings of annoyance by, in effect, battering her husband. In these days in which battering of relatives is so often in the headlines I expect to read before long that some non-sleeping wife has actually gone ahead and done this. If so, I hope the court takes the view that she acted under extreme provocation. Snoring is more likely to happen when you are sleeping on your back as in this position you often breathe through your mouth. It may have had some advantages in primitive man, for when you are lying on your back sleeping you are an easy target for an attacking animal. But the noise some make when snoring is enough to frighten the bravest of animals.

(Don't tell your snoring husband this because he will only start boasting about it.) If you can persuade the snorer to breathe through his nose again you might be lucky and the habit will stop. There are many medical troubles that block up noses and lead to snoring. In children swollen adenoids are a common cause of mouth-breathing and snoring. These little glands are at the back of the nose and can block up the airway entirely. Sinus infection and injuries to the nose can do the same. These conditions can and should be treated, not because snoring is dangerous, but because they can cause more damage if left untreated.

You will notice that I am assuming most snorers are men. This is probably true, although many women snore as well. Somehow their snoring is not so loud as men's and does not cause the same problems. Men would claim that as insomnia is commoner in women they complain about snoring more, so you can argue both ways. Treating the snorer is not easy, but you might start with an Anti-Snore Ball, which can be bought and sewn on to the back of the pajama trousers. Every time he turns on his back the discomfort of the ball encourages him to turn over on his side again. With luck, he breathes through his nose and the problem is solved. Others are less lucky, and mouth-breathing continues in every position. For them, special masks can be bought which stretch over the chin and face, completely shutting off the mouth so that they are forced to breathe through their noses. Others only snore in deep sleep and a sharp prod in the ribs or back may be all that is sufficient to bring them up a stage or two in sleep so that they stop snoring. The best advice I can give to their sleeping partners is to get a good set of ear-plugs.

What is the purpose of sleep? It may seem odd for a state in which we spend one-third of our lives, but we still do not really know. It appears to be necessary for all but the simplest of animals and serves a restorative purpose, best expressed in the words of that keen observer of human psychology, William Shakespeare: 'sleep that knits up the raveled sleeve of care, the death of each day's life, sore labor's bath, balm of hurt minds, great nature's second course, chief nourisher in life's feast'. Four centuries later we add little more. It has recently been discovered that during orthodox (non-REM) sleep one of the hormones necessary for a healthy body-growth hormone-passes into the bloodstream. Growth hormone is essential for growth in children but continues to be needed in adult life. The body, like a building buffeted by wind and rain, needs regular maintenance if it is to work well. Growth hormone helps in this maintenance, speeding up the production of new cells to replace old and dying ones, strengthening bone, building muscle and supporting tissues. There is some evidence that prolonged sleeplessness in children (which usually has a physical or environmental cause rather than an emotional one) can hold back growth because not enough growth hormone is produced.

The feeling of well-being and refreshment that follows sound sleep is at least partly due to growth hormone having performed its task well.

The purpose of REM sleep is less certain. As mentioned earlier, some authorities think that there is a need to dream in the same way as there is a need to sleep, and that the many changes that take place in the REM phase of sleep are all by-products of dreaming.

This of course begs the question: why should there be a need to dream? Another view is that whereas orthodox sleep restores bodily function, REM sleep restores brain function. The brain is different from most other organs in the body in that nerve cells do not get replaced when they die, so there is not the same turnover as in other parts of the body. Nevertheless, the brain still needs maintenance and repair, and during REM sleep there is an increased blood flow to the nerve cells, freeing them of waste products and increasing efficiency. This, by the way, tends to support the 'vacuum cleaner' theory of dreaming.

There is evidence that the brain is better at learning if this is carried out immediately before sleep. When the hard-pressed student stays up late revising before an examination, the next morning he is likely to retain more of this knowledge than if he goes to bed and wakes up early, and then starts his revision. Some of this improved efficiency is also due to the relative absence of stimuli reaching the brain during sleep so that what you learn has a better chance of being retained. Some lazy minds have had the idea that learning may also take place during sleep, an idea popularized in Aldous Huxley's novel *Brave New World.* In this science-fiction story, education started early. Children were taught from babyhood by playing tape-recordings over and over again during sleep till they remembered every word. This sleep teaching, or hypnopaedia, as it was called, concentrated on moral education, convincing each child that its position in the social structure was more favorable than those of others. Unfortunately for the student, but fortunately for those who value their freedoms, learning cannot take place while we are asleep. The brain cannot discriminate between learning stimuli and irrelevant ones and clamps down on all of them. So please ignore those appealing advertisements that claim that learning can take place in sleep and offer equipment at exorbitant prices for this purpose. The claims are nonsense.

Further support for the idea that REM sleep is concerned with maintenance of the brain comes from the pattern of sleep at different ages. Very young children up to the age of two spend a much greater amount of time in REM sleep than older children or adults. The brain is actively growing during the first two years of life and has the greatest number of nerve cells. From two onwards the number gets steadily fewer (but the capacity to learn is still great as many of the cells remain unused or underemployed). As the increase in REM sleep coincides with active growth in the brain, it seems likely that the two are related.

There may be argument about the purpose of sleep but there is none about the, need. Both types of sleep are needed and the body and brain have their own internal methods of ensuring this. For a large number of body functions a balance is maintained by automatic feedback mechanisms. For example, the amount of water in the body is kept within remarkably constant limits. If we drink too little fluid the kidneys concentrate the urine so that less fluid is lost. We then feel thirsty and drink more.

If we drink too much fluid the kidneys allow more urine to be got rid of until the excess load is removed. Most of these mechanisms do not involve us in any conscious awareness-they go on automatically all the time. This complex balancing act also occurs with sleep. If we have too little orthodox sleep one night we will have more on the next night to make up for it. If we have poor orthodox sleep for two nights we make up the extra sleep on the third night, with possibly a carry-over to the fourth. It is as though there was a sleep debt which has to be made up to keep the balance. A similar pattern occurs with REM sleep. Experiments have been done with people in sleep laboratories who have been woken whenever their brain waves and behaviour show that they are coming into REM sleep. Subsequently these people spend a much greater part of their sleep in the REM phase until the 'REM debt' is made up. Now, as an insomniac, you may well ask, what use is this information to me? You must think that your balancing mechanisms are not working; otherwise you would not have the problem of continual sleeplessness.

After a night without sleep you have another night without sleep, and never seem to make it up. In one sense this is true, at least for those insomniacs who genuinely have fewer than five hours' sleep nightly, but even in these people compensatory mechanisms are working to make lack of sleep less of a problem. As we noted earlier, the deepest stages of sleep are achieved within three hours of falling asleep. The old saying 'an hour's sleep before midnight is worth two afterwards' reflects this; the first hours of sleep are the most valuable. If you become deprived of sleep on one night you spend longer in the deepest stage of sleep on the next night, and even if the total number of sleep hours is still too small, you will have had a greater proportion of sound sleep than if you had slept well the previous night. Insomniacs may find it hard to credit this, but please let me emphasize again that it is the sleep you miss that you remember, not the sleep you have. And, finally, could I also add a few words to the husband or wife of the insomniac which should have become apparent from this chapter.

Remember at night when you are lying next to your apparently sleepless spouse that if he or she chatters idly from time to time, jerks occasionally, apparently wakes and looks around like a hunted animal, changes sleeping position twenty to thirty times in the course of the night and displays amorous intentions at regular intervals, these are not necessarily ways of overcoming the boredom and frustration of those sleepless hours. These actions may have woken you, but your partner may have been sleeping soundly all the time.

The Effects of Too Little Sleep

What happens when you have too little sleep? In answering this question we have to separate effects from causes. Because a problem is associated with insomnia it is not necessarily caused by it. To start with we have to exclude those who claim to be short of sleep but in fact have eight or nine hours of sleep each night. Even after excluding these people there is still some difficulty in deciding when an individual is becoming deprived of sleep.

This is because of the great range of sleeping habits between different people. Old sayings about sleep, such as 'six hours for a man, eight for a woman and nine for a fool', and 'nature requires five, custom takes seven, laziness takes nine and wickedness eleven', have no basis.

There is also an important relationship between age and sleep. On average an infant of two months sleeps for eighteen hours a day, a three-year-old toddler for thirteen hours, a twenty-five-year-old adult for eight hours and a seventy-five-year-old for five hours a day. These differences are not explained merely by evidence, for example, that the elderly have more insomnia. They indicate that at different times of development the body needs differing amounts of sleep. For anyone person it is impossible to decide what is the right number of hours of sleep and the obsession that many have with the figure of eight hours is quite unnecessary, reflecting the common need to put limits on things that are indefinable.

One way of finding out the effects of too little sleep is to take people not suffering from insomnia and deprive them of sleep for varying periods of time. As one might expect, this can only be done with volunteers. In extreme cases the person is prevented from going to sleep for as long as possible and is shaken awake each time he shows signs of dropping off ..Most of us have little difficulty in staying awake for twenty-four hours but after this time problems arise. Unless you constantly change your level of stimulation you quickly drift into sleep. It is the change in the stimulation that matters, not how strong it is. It is easy for sleep-deprived people to fall asleep in the presence of blinding white light or music played at maximum volume on a record player, but it is more difficult when the white light is replaced by a variable flickering with colors of different intensities or when the music alternates between jazz, pop and classical music.

As time goes on and you become sleepier, even changes in stimulation are ignored. For example, you might think that a country walk was an exercise that would inhibit sleep. There are changes in sight, sound, touch and smell, and you often hear the adjectives 'bracing' and 'stimulating' applied to this activity. None-the-less it is quite possible for a sleep-deprived person to fall asleep while walking, even to continue the correct movements as if he was still awake. It is as though the higher parts of the brain had closed down all contact with the lower parts while the latter continued to function normally. The person is literally sleep-walking, although the circumstances differ from most forms of somnambulism.

Before excessive tiredness is noticed by the subject he has greater difficulty in carrying out certain jobs, particularly those which are monotonous. The ability to maintain the constant level of alertness over a long period is called vigilance and is particularly affected by shortage of sleep. There are many tasks which require vigilance (e.g. checking machinery which is in continuous operation) and apart from the likelihood of falling asleep during the task the person is less likely to detect the changes that require some action to correct them. Concentration is also affected when sleep lack has occurred; the mind wanders and efficiency

is impaired.

In real life the person who is short of sleep usually realizes that he is not doing his work as well as he does normally. This leads to a conscious effort to work harder and make up for the inefficiency. This extra effort works up to a point, but only at the cost of irritability and other symptoms such as headaches. The person is more easily distracted by noise and other interruptions, and in trying to overcome them the headaches get worse, tension increases, efficiency gets less and he ends up in a state of exhaustion. This situation is similar to a typist having to wear gloves and dark spectacles during her work. At first she can overcome the handicap by concentrating harder but the compensation will not last long and exactly the   vicious cycle of shortage of sleep-inefficiency-increased effort -tension symptoms--exhaustion leading to further inefficiency, can only be broken by having a good sleep.

Of course symptoms such as tension, irritability and headaches are not always caused by insomnia and, indeed, it is people who tend to have these symptoms anyway who often have trouble with sleeping. But insomnia would definitely make them worse.

In more severe sleep deprivation peculiar things happen. These changes rarely occur in real-life insomnia because they only happen when shortage of sleep is very severe. At this stage people will fall asleep no matter where they are or what they are doing and it is only when forced to keep active or encouraged to talk that they will stay awake. Because the need to sleep is so strong, not even the most hardened insomniac can resist dropping off at this stage.

So really severe sleep deprivation is only seen under artificial conditions after about sixty hours without sleep.

At this stage the senses begin to play tricks. Voices sound as though they are made in an echo chamber, or a squeak may sound like a roar. Light and shade get confused and the imagination runs riot. Strange figures and shapes are seen which are mistaken for real people and objects. The person feels detached and unreal and often gets the peculiar impression that he is standing outside his body and that his mind is working on its own. He reels around as though he is drunk. He may feel that other people are against him and are threatening to harm him in some way.

He confuses night and day and cannot remember familiar faces. It is like a dream or nightmare except that he is still awake. These experiences may last for many hours and if sleep is still prevented some harm can result. Even after a few days of normal sleeping these ideas often persist and may take many weeks to disappear entirely. The experiences are not particularly pleasant, but I doubt whether any insomniac reading this has ever had any of them to a significant extent. The effects of sleep lack tell us how important sleep is to the body, but the rarity with which these really strange feelings occur also tells us how efficient the body is in making up lost sleep. So remember this the next time you are telling somebody you have not had a good sleep for over twenty years.

Why Don't You Go to Sleep?

Worry is perhaps the biggest single factor behind sleeplessness. Almost everyone has had mild insomnia at some time, usually associated with worry. This is particularly common the night before a big occasion like moving house, an important interview, examinations, or a hospital operation. Thoughts about the problem have recurred time and time again the day before the occasion-an unpleasant round that never seems to end. You hope that you will feel better after a good night's sleep but, no, when you go to bed the thoughts still go on endlessly. There is no solution to them; it is not the same as concentrating on a problem which has one or more correct answers.

There is no answer but you cannot stop thinking about it. The more painful the worry, the more you try and forget it and the less successful you will be. Your brain waves are fast and active and the slow, quiet waves of sleep do not get a look in. Your bed, which before was always inviting, warm and cosy, no longer seems a friendly place.

You come across bumps and hollows which you had never noticed before, no place is comfortable and you change your position over and over again. You are easily distracted by the noise of traffic and flashes of light, and by the wind sighing in the eaves or the sound of a train in the night.

In this very frequent type of sleeplessness the worrying is always about something real and relevant. It is reasonable to be concerned whether the removal men will lose or break any of your cherished possessions when you move house the next day, although staying awake and worrying will not help matters. Insomnia related to this type of worry is soon over, and the event passes and all is well again. Long-term worry leads to chronic insomnia and here the problems are much more complicated. Again there may be worry about a real problem, such as illness in the family, work or money troubles, which are unlikely to be sorted out in a few days. Too much responsibility often leads to worry. For many, nothing could be more worrying than the responsibility of running a country, a worry that led to chronic insomnia in Lord Rosebery, prime minister in the UK at the end of the nineteenth century. Faced with the alternatives of continuing as a sleepless prime minister or resigning, he chose the latter, and slept well again.

Long-term worries return night after night and frequently during the day as well. Whenever the mind is unoccupied they fill the gap, so it is hardly surprising that they are such a trouble just before going to sleep. When the problem causing the worry is removed the insomnia usually gets better as well, although there is always the danger that once the sleepless pattern has become ingrained it will not alter.

There are other worries about real problems which are not so easily resolved. Thoughts and doubts of death and the afterlife, the meaning of existence and the powers of the supernatural can grind on continuously in the mind.

They are problems that concern us all, but for most they are put on one side, conveniently suppressed despite their importance. For some they demand an answer, even though the mind is incapable of giving one, and sleeplessness is the result. Often these ideas are realized to be pointless, useless or ridiculous, but despite conscious effort to be rid of them the person still finds himself forced to think about them. Doctors call these ideas obsessional ruminations and they can be important in insomnia.

Moving on from real worries we come to 'imaginary fears'. I put this in inverted commas because the term is not really true; the fears are real enough but they are fears about things which should not make us afraid. They include fears about physical health (in the absence of physical illness), fears about losing consciousness and control, and of dying in the night from suffocation or a similar unpleasant end. Unjustified worries about health are the key features of hypochondriacs and there are few of us who can claim that our lives are completely free of them.

The hypochondriac lying in bed at night is all too conscious of every change in his bodily functions. He hears his breathing, is aware of his heart beating, feels his stomach rumbling, his ears popping, joints twinging and muscles contracting. Any unexpected change, such as, for example, his heart missing a beat (which is fairly common and quite healthy), is liable to reinforce the fear of serious disease and set in motion a chain of worry. Having medical check-ups and tests which show no evidence of disease is not enough to satisfy health fears and at night they are often at their most rampant.

Fears about losing consciousness with the feeling that you are no longer in control of your life can also be a problem. Just before dropping off to sleep you go through a phase of dozing when you feel your mind slipping into blackness and oblivion. The same feeling is also experienced when having a general anesthetic in hospital and some people find it pleasant.

Recently it has become a fashion among some young people to get to this state of partial consciousness because it gives them a kick. They deliberately try to bring it on by taking drugs or similar means, but people like this make up a small minority. A few find the feeling extremely unpleasant, and instead of drifting off to sleep naturally at night they are jerked to full wakefulness in a panic when they notice this sensation. It appears to be frightening because during sleep you are more defenseless than at any other time.

The famous children's writer, Hans Christian Andersen, feared for much of his life that other people might think he was dead when he was sleeping. He had an intense fear of closed spaces (claustrophobia) and was particularly afraid that he might be sealed in a coffin while sleeping and wake to find himself unable to escape. He therefore made a point of carrying a notice with him wherever he went. It read 'I am not dead, I am only sleeping', and he would hang this at the foot of his bed each night.

Fears of dying in the night are quite common and can cause insomnia. In fact there is no evidence that death occurs more commonly during the sleeping hours than at other times and the fear of dying in a panic, struggling to get your breath, seldom turns out to be true. It arises because some nervous people often wake in the night feeling that they cannot get their breath although they are physically well. Severe panic can be associated with difficulties in breathing. However it seems to the person going through the experience, the panic comes first and the breathing troubles afterwards and there is no danger of dying. The one exception is in some people with heart disease, whom we shall come to later.

The more that worries about imaginary rather than real dangers are behind insomnia, the more likely are they to be associated with mental disorder. Insomnia is very frequently part of a mental disorder although many would prefer to think that they just had insomnia and nothing else.

There are still a number of false ideas about the nature of mental disorder which need correcting. Many years ago the only mental disorders that were recognized were severe forms of illness that led to admission to a mental hospital. Today we realize that mental disorder covers a much broader range, including emotional problems in ordinary people. The threatening statement 'you ought to go and see a psychiatrist' carries with it the undertones that you are mad and don't realize it and need some form of treatment. In fact, most of the people who see psychiatrists are only too well aware that they are not well. They come for help because of unpleasant feelings, feelings that they usually succeed in keeping from others and therefore seem quite well.

Most of the mental disorders associated with insomnia come into this group, which together make up the neuroses. Unfortunately the word 'neurotic' has acquired qualities which were not originally intended. The idea that someone with a neurosis is 'putting it on', exaggerating symptoms and is really quite well but won't admit it, is quite wrong. A person with a neurosis has something wrong and although it may be less tangible than the handicap associated with a broken leg it is none-the-less real.

Medical language is only convenient shorthand for communication between doctors. Names of mental disorders are part of this language, neither more nor less, and certainly not terms of criticism or abuse. In general medicine the special words that doctors use can be reassuring.

You may have heard of a person who goes to his doctor with a heavy cold, is examined briefly and told by the doctor that he has coryza. He leaves the surgery feeling much better now that the doctor has diagnosed his condition, particularly if he also has a prescription for some special medicine. In fact the doctor has done nothing more than repeat what the patient knows already, as coryza is the technical name for the virus infection causing the symptoms of a cold. Yet if a nervous person with insomnia goes to a doctor and is told that he has an anxiety neurosis he may feel annoyed because this sounds like a criticism. But although you may feel that 'anxiety neurosis' is a less comfortable label than 'coryza', the same process is working in both cases, translating everyday language into medical jargon. In any case the line that divides 'neurosis' from 'normal' is not a fixed one so you should not feel there is any special significance if you fall on one side rather than the other. Doctors fix this line by finding out how severe are the symptoms and how much suffering is caused by them, and not whether they dislike the person concerned or have got out of the wrong side of the bed that morning.

There are many neuroses that can cause insomnia. Anxiety neuroses (or states) are among the most common.

Try imagining how you felt at some time in the past when you were extremely frightened. Your body must have reacted very strongly; your mouth went dry, your heart thumped away in your chest like a sledgehammer, your muscles became tense and rigid, and you felt like screaming or running away. You felt threatened by something terrible and your mind worked overtime trying to find a solution to the problem. You may think that the changes that occurred in your body when you were anxious were just unpleasant feelings of no possible value. They probably were of no value to you at the time, but if you were about to be attacked by a wild animal the changes in your body would have helped you in getting away from the danger as quickly as possible. Unfortunately the person with an anxiety state has no obvious danger to escape from. The unpleasant feelings of anxiety are there all the time, even at night when he should be relaxing and going to sleep. His mind is like a tense spring which cannot. unwind, and going to sleep is a process taking many hours.

Depression is also behind many cases of insomnia. In its most common form, the natural depression that follows an unpleasant event such as the death of a relative leads to morbid thoughts that preoccupy the mind when you should be ready for sleep. Try as you may, every time you try and think of something else only gloom can be seen.

I doubt whether anyone reading this has never had a night when sad thoughts have prevented normal sleep, and, indeed, they are part of the normal process of mourning. It is only when they persist for many weeks that the depression becomes abnormal and outside help may be needed.

The most serious form of insomnia is found with certain types of depression. In these cases the depressed person has no trouble getting off to sleep, but wakes in the early hours of the morning. When he wakes the whole future seems black and hopeless. He cannot get off to sleep again and often gets out of bed in the hope that he can rid his mind of gloomy thoughts. But they persist and he lies awake for hours before dozing off into a fitful sleep. The feelings of depression may be so strong that thoughts of suicide come to mind, and it is a sad fact that many successful suicides take place in the early hours of the morning.

The fears about health we mentioned earlier are also common in depressed people. Minor health problems are thought of as serious illnesses with a fatal outcome. The motto of the depressive seems to be 'the worst always happens' so every little pain and ache is exaggerated to mean impending death. When someone is severely depressed with these fears it is no use trying to convince them that the thoughts are silly and unnecessary. Of course the healthy person knows that they are stupid, and the sleepless hours thinking about them are spent to no good purpose, but it takes more than words to convince them otherwise. To us the fears and worries are imagination; to the depressed person they are real. To alter them requires changing the person's whole outlook on the world and a doctor's help is often required.

Finally we should mention some people who are not really anxious or depressed but who are chronic worriers. If they do not have something to worry about they will make up something. They are often quite at home with their old familiar worries; it is new ones that concern them more. Try thinking about possible reasons for worrying and you can come up with dozens, but most of us accept that life is too short to get worked up about them. Our chronic worrier plans everything for months ahead and not only crosses his bridges before he comes to them but expects each of them to collapse under him. Such people can easily cotton on to insomnia as a cause of worry. They plan their eight hours' sleep nightly like a military maneuver and if they only get seven and a half they feel cheated. They do not realize that the human frame is flexible and can make up for a few lost hours of sleep, and so a chain of worry begins. Some of these people are phony insomniacs, convincing themselves they are short of sleep but actually getting more than the average. They seek help repeatedly but are never satisfied by what is given, which is hardly surprising as there is no sleep disturbance to treat.

Many suffer from insomnia when their sleep routine changes. Rhythms of activity are present in all animals and plants but it is only recently that we have realized how much they influence human lives. Unfortunately modern man is expected to change his pattern of life repeatedly, one day working for twelve hours doing vigorous exercise, the next engaged in mental effort with no physical activity, and every so often having a relaxing day doing nothing. The sleep rhythm usually copes well with these changes but it can fail. This often happens in shift workers when they change from night to day work and vice versa. Although they quickly adjust to working again at the new time, it is not so easy to get back to normal sleep. This is because the sleep rhythm needs time to readjust, chemical changes have to take place and these are not to be hurried. So if you continue working as though nothing had happened after a change of shift you are liable to get insomnia, to feel irritable and bad-tempered while awake, and to be less efficient at making decisions. Employers now realize these difficulties, which can become real dangers if you drive or work with complicated machinery, and allow a few days to readjust when there is a change of shift. Exactly the same problem occurs in long-distance air flights. It is now possible to take off from

London in the morning and arrive in New York at an earlier time on the same morning, even though the flight has taken several hours. The reason for this is not that you have been travelling backwards in time, but that you have crossed several time zones, each one being earlier than the one you have left. The effect of this is the same as changing a work shift. You get out of the aircraft after a full day's flying but instead of taking a well-earned sleep you have to face another day. By the time night comes you cannot sleep because your rhythms have been put out of joint, and you show all the symptoms of jet lag. This special form of insomnia is predictable and is easily overcome within a few days by taking sleep when it is needed and avoiding stress.

You should take more notice of your biological clock than of the manmade clocks all around you.

Insomnia caused by much smaller changes in sleep pattern is very common. Some people insist they cannot sleep properly away from the comfort and security of their own bedrooms. They have carefully planned lives in which any change can be upsetting. They retire to bed at the same time each night and are very fussy about the nightclothes they wear, the temperature of the bedroom, the color and texture of the sheets and the number of blankets. A small alteration, such as a yellow sheet instead of a white one, fills them with alarm, and they cannot sleep until the sheet is changed. I t is no wonder that moving to a new sleeping place, whether it is a hotel, ship or another house, is too great a change for them. In one sense these stay-at-homes are right. It takes time to adapt to a new sleep setting and often there is insomnia on the first night in the new place. But as we said earlier, once you have become used to it, there is no problem over sleep. It will take longer to adapt to unpleasant sleeping conditions than pleasant ones but it will happen eventually. This is why mountain climbers can sleep roped together high on an exposed rock face, why horse-riders can sleep in the saddle, and why ordinary folk can sleep all night on cold, bare pavements to be the first in the queue for the January sales. Too many think they cannot sleep in strange places but would be surprised at their ability to do so. I have come across people who would not consider travelling on a sleeper train overnight but who regularly drop off when making their half-hour commuter trip each morning and evening. If the only thing stopping you from staying with relatives, taking a holiday or travelling abroad is concern about your sleep, then go ahead and make plans to leave.

It may take a day or so to catch up, but your sleep will soon look after itself.

Your physical health may have a lot to do with insomnia. At its simplest level, the right balance between physical and mental exercise is an aid to good sleeping.

We need ordinary sleep to restore the body, and REM sleep to restore the mind, and it is much better for sound sleep to have these needs balanced. We are often told how a life of continuous mental activity or brain work is harmful for us, but continuous physical exertion can have the same effect. The expression 'I was so tired I could not sleep' illustrates this; exhaustion does not mean that healthy sleep will follow. Of course striking the balance between exercise and rest, work and play, mind and body, is not only important for good sleep but good health all round, so there are plenty of reasons for getting this part of your life in order.

Of the physical illnesses that cause trouble with sleeping it is those that cause pain that are most troublesome. I have pointed out how adaptable the body and mind are to changes, even changes that are unpleasant. This is why it is possible to sleep in the most uncomfortable places.

When you first lie on a lumpy apple-pie bed your brain gets hundreds of messages from your skin and muscles which all tell you to go away and find something more comfortable to lie on. If you ignore these signals the messages get less and less. The sensitive parts of your body get less sensitive. You get used to that nasty lump poking into the middle of your back and the lump soon feels almost cozy. This marvelous ability to get used to

discomfort even extends to pain, but only if it comes from outside the body. The fakir who lies on his bed of nails feels most uncomfortable to begin with. A thousand little needles bore into his skin, but if he is careful not to move too much his body gets accustomed to the pricks, and the pain gradually goes.

If it was the same for internal pain, pain coming from inside the body, a great deal of suffering and insomnia would be prevented. But such pain does not get less with the passage of time. The opposite often happens, the pain gets worse and worse and the sufferer has to do something drastic to help it. Pain often seems more severe when there is nothing else to occupy the mind. Sleep is a merciful release from the pain as well as a need in its own right. If insomnia is caused by pain, every attempt should be made to relieve the pain before other ways of helping sleep are tried. Backache is a common source of pain, and this can often be helped by sleeping on a hard mattress or by having boards underneath. Other pains may also be worse when lying down. They include some stomach disorders and ulcers and often the sufferer feels better when propped up in bed with several pillows. There is no special reason why you should sleep lying down, although it is the usual custom nowadays. The Vikings used to sleep sitting up and fully dressed in very short beds, and insomnia did not seem to trouble them too much. In times of emergency they were quickly out of bed and a fighting force in no time, so their sleeping habits had advantages.

Patients with heart disease often need to sleep propped up in bed as well. This prevents their lungs from getting too congested so they can breathe more easily during sleep. Hospital beds are adjustable and can be altered to any level, and many ill patients sleep with their bodies raised as well. If you have ever tried sleeping on a slope you will usually find it is more comfortable having your head at the top and your feet at the bottom. The ritual of having your bed completely flat is an unnecessary one, so do not let it bother you if you have to sleep in an unusual position.

Coughing over and over again can also stop you from sleeping, and this may also occur more often at night when you are lying flat. Fluid draining from the tubes and passages in your nose and face, particularly the sinuses, can irritate the chest and lead to bouts of coughing.

There is nothing worse than lying in bed trying not to cough when you want to. You end up with an explosive splutter, which not only wakes you up completely but often wakes everyone else in the room as well. Taking the opposite line of coughing when you feel like it also does not help. Each cough tends to make you cough more till your throat feels as though it is on fire. The right thing to do is to take a cough linctus or something similar which will temporarily suppress the cough and allow you to get to sleep. This is no substitute for treating the cause of the cough as well; so do not rely on your linctus alone.

If physical illness causes insomnia, then it is the illness that should be treated, not the insomnia. It is only when the treatment for the illness is unsuccessful or only partly relieves the condition that the insomnia may need to be treated as well. Unfortunately there are still a large number of medical illnesses that can cause insomnia and which can only be partly helped by modern treatments.

Arthritis is perhaps the commonest of these and again it is pain that prevents sleep. Once the pain is relieved sleep should follow, but we lack the universal pain-killer that is always effective. Some of these types of insomnia may only respond to sleeping tablets and we shall come across these later.

Self-help for Insomnia

By now you will have realized whether or not you are an insomniac. If you are, you will want to know how to sleep well again. The first stage is to find out the likely causes of your difficulty in sleeping. We have already discussed many of the causes of insomnia in the previous chapter, and you may have identified the one that is stopping you from sleeping. More likely you will have found several possible causes, some of which you can do something about, and others which seem insoluble. It is just possible that you have not found anything in this book so far which helps you to find out what is causing your difficulty in sleeping. If this is the case with you, I want you to think very carefully before sitting back smugly and thinking that you have defied the pundits and produced sleeplessness out of nowhere. It is more likely that you have not admitted to yourself that there are problems in your life, problems which can be obscured but not buried completely. Is your life as settled and secure as you make it out to be? Are you really contented and fulfilled in your work, in your spiritual life, and in your relationships with others, of both sexes?

Are you really being honest with yourself? Try and answer these questions before moving on to the practical issue of treating your insomnia.

If the causes of your insomnia cannot be changed, then it is fair to consider treating it directly. But this is never as good as removing the cause itself. It is much easier to treat your insomnia than to take a big step such as giving up your job and trying something completely new, a change which is full of risks but at least is likely to give you peace of mind. In this day and age we are impatient for instant solutions to our problems, solutions which involve us in the minimum of effort. In the long term, our instant solutions may do more harm than good, so always treat them with caution.

Self-help should always be tried first in dealing with insomnia. Much of it will be seen as common-sense advice in view of our knowledge of normal sleep, but it may be more effective than more specialized treatments. You have to bear in mind all those things which tend to make us sleepy, even at times when we should be awake. They include warmth, relaxation, lack of sleep, boredom, food, security and familiarity. If you are not getting to sleep when you should, try and alter your sleeping pattern and behavior so that all these things are present at the time you go to bed.

Warmth is very important. It takes longer to get off to sleep in a cold bed in a cold room than it does in a warm, cozy bed. Some people still have the idea that it is healthy to sleep in a cold bedroom with the window open to let in the raw night air. This is quite untrue, and such habits can be actually harmful to health if you suffer from bronchitis and other chest complaints. A warm atmosphere does not do any harm, provided there is adequate ventilation between rooms, and it certainly aids sleep. A warm bed is even more important and provided you have the right bedclothes your own body makes enough heat to make the bed warm. When you first go to bed it can feel chilly and uninviting. So particularly if your bedroom is cold, a hot-water bottle or electric blanket may help.

Taking a hot bath or shower before going to bed on cold nights will also warm you up and help you to relax. Too much warmth, of course, can prevent sleep, and on hot, sticky nights those who have no air-conditioning in their bedrooms are very envious of those who have.

Relaxation is easier to write about than to achieve, and we shall come across this again later. But as well as helping your body and mind to relax you can help by having a comfortable bed that is a pleasure to sleep in. Choosing the right mattress and bed is most important. It has to be a personal choice; a bed that is heavenly for one may be hell to another and, provided the two do not intend sleeping in the same bed, the choice should not be too difficult. It will involve testing the product and not just taking for granted the smooth words in the glossy brochures telling you of all the latest gimmicks that have made a bed the most 'slumberful' yet. Your mind may believe it, but your body is less easily persuaded. So test the bed by lying on it, rolling over, taking up your various sleeping positions, and see how you feel. Make sure the bed is the right length and width. For those over six feet in height, many beds are too short. Tell the salesman, who gets a commission on the sale and will often do anything to sell the bed, to go away and come back in fifteen minutes, so you have enough time to make your decision. You cannot decide whether a bed is comfortable when someone is hovering over you like a bird of prey. Buying a bed is a long-term investment for the future which should not be made too lightly.

Once you have your comfortable bed and mattress you have a wide range of sheets, blankets, pillows, quilts and eiderdowns to choose from. Again there are no hard and fast rules in making your choice. In recent years there has been a move away from thick, heavy blankets to light, airy quilts, although in Scandinavia they have used quilts (or duvets) for many years. The warmest and lightest quilts are those filled with goose down (closely followed by duck down and feathers), but synthetic filling materials are improving year by year and are almost as good. When choosing a quilt make sure that you are not allergic to the filling material, or you may end up with a new cause for insomnia, a persistent sneeze, running nose and sore eyes.

Also check the filling in the pillows for the same reason.

If you choose blankets, there is no reason to feel a stick-in- the-mud. Many prefer the tighter feeling that they give and as they are tucked in under the mattress you feel more secure. The important thing is to have a bed that is warm and comfortable, and in which you feel at home.

The bedroom is also important. Some people prefer certain colors in their bedroom decor as they find them restful and relaxing. The color varies from person to person, and the old idea that one color, it used to be green, was the most soporific, has been abandoned.

Choose the colors you like and remember when the lights are out all colors look the same. The position of the bed also seems to be important for many people. Some want it near a window, others prefer it in a dark corner, and most will have it placed against at least one wall. This seems to be related to the sense of security that walls bring. People feel exposed and nervous sleeping in the middle of a room, even though it may be more convenient for the bed to be placed there. Others insist that they only sleep well if they lie in the plane of the rotation of the earth, or along the magnetic lines of force. We have to face it: insomnia has led to some very cranky ideas.

What you wear in bed also depends on personal wishes.

Some always prefer to sleep naked, others need three layers of clothing before settling down for the night. Some prefer the feel of nylon, others find cotton more comforting, and many prefer the feel of another warm body. Not long ago it was thought to be unhygienic to sleep in the same bed as somebody else. I do not know on what evidence this statement was made, and suspect it stemmed more from Victorian modesty and prudishness than from anything else. Certainly the twelve members of the sixteenth-century family in the town of Ware in Hertfordshire who all slept in the same bed did not appear to suffer from more disease than their contemporaries.

Their bed, which came to be known as the Great Bed of Ware, was nearly eleven feet square and almost nine feet tall. As the bed was square the family had the choice of sleeping with their heads at any of the four sides and often slept with six each at opposite ends of the bed. In the historical accounts of the use of the bed there is no mention of insomnia. Although the bed became famous and was even mentioned by Shakespeare in one of his plays, the idea of large beds did not catch on. Our cave living ancestors used to sleep in groups for reasons of warmth and safety. They lay in a circle with their feet towards the fire, which gave them protection during the night. This way of sleeping must have given a great sense of security and togetherness.

Nowadays it is uncommon for more than two to sleep in a bed, and the two are usually of different sexes and are already intimate. Sleeping in a double bed may produce insomnia if your partner snores, thrashes about the bed in the night, sleep-talks or sleep-walks, or happens to be one of those people who takes up the whole bed.

Some have this ability to fill up all the bed space available and their partners are left curled up at one edge, often lacking blankets or sheets, feeling cold, miserable and irritated.

Attempts to retrieve their rightful share of the bed and bedclothes are met with violent pummeling, pushing and twisting movements until they are back where they started. Even if the unfortunate sufferer does drop off to sleep, their position at the edge of the bed is so precarious that they are in danger of falling off while asleep. If you happen to sleep in a double bed with someone who will not give you a fair share of the accommodation you will be well advised to go back to sleeping in a single bed. It is no use arguing with your partner, he or she will be as sweet as pie when awake and promise all you ask, but once asleep it is quite a different story. There is something of the cuckoo make-up in his personality, the nest will not be shared and he is only happy when he has it to himself.

On the other hand there are those who sleep much better with someone in a double bed. The sound of someone sleeping peacefully and breathing regularly beside you is very soporific, and indeed, some enterprising manufacturers of sleep-aids have produced models that imitate this sound. The warmth of somebody next to you is also soothing and is better than the best hot-water bottle as it stays at just the right temperature. Such people only get insomnia when they have to sleep on their own for short periods. There is a feeling of security that many get from sleeping close to another in a double bed. The frightened crying child who cannot get to sleep in his own bed will drop off immediately if he is allowed to share his parents' bed for a few minutes. He no longer feels frightened because he feels protected and safe. We still have similar feelings as adults, which explains why so many feel more settled in a double bed.

The relationship between sex and insomnia is complex, and inevitably comes up when discussing the advantages and disadvantages of double beds. As we said earlier, relaxation aids sleep and there is no doubt that mutually satisfying sexual intercourse before sleep can help insomnia. If both man and woman reach orgasm, that is ejaculation of sperm in the male, and rhythmic movements of the sexual organs (particularly the vagina and clitoris) in the female, then both will be relaxed and prepared for sleep. There are many different forms of sexual response and they have to be understood if sex is not to lead to insomnia. If either partner just fails to reach orgasm, the sexual act becomes frustrating and anything but relaxing. While one partner slumbers peacefully the other lies sexually aroused but unsatisfied, and this does no good for sleep. Some take over an hour before they are ready for intercourse while others become aroused immediately. Women in general take longer to be aroused than men, although there are many exceptions and the difference is now realized to be less than was once thought. Although we are living in a world where sex is openly advertised and exploited, many are still too shy to talk about sexual matters within marriage.

Men who can discuss in detail with other men techniques of intercourse while lecherously looking at a photograph in a sex magazine show no inclination to talk about the same subject with their wives. If there is no proper communication between husband and wife at this level then sex is bound to give rise to problems, and this will not help insomnia. At its simplest level many couples are not able to tell each other when they want intercourse, so the clumsy leap in the bed becomes the first indication.

If you are too embarrassed to talk openly about this you can develop special cues or signs which can be ignored or replied to without feelings being hurt. There should be no misunderstanding when the couple go to bed, one thinking the other is ready for intercourse and the other thinking the opposite. This is a recipe for trouble and if it goes on they will soon be sleeping in single beds again.

Sex should not be thought of as a cure for insomnia. A healthy sex life is part of good life adjustment but it need not be part of a pre-sleep ritual. If it interferes with sleep, then you should choose a different time for intercourse.

One time when sex is particularly likely to interfere with sleep is in the middle of the night, when one partner, usually the man, wakes up with strong sexual urges, wakes his wife and forces intercourse while she is still only half awake. He then goes off to sleep again while she stays awake, frustrated and annoyed, and takes a long time to get off to sleep again. This is male chauvinism at its worst and shows no consideration for the feelings of the woman.

Lack of sleep itself is a powerful cure for insomnia. This may seem an obvious statement, but it is often forgotten.

For example, there are those who are so obsessed by their sleep rituals that they always go to bed at the same time each night whether they feel sleepy or not. The ritual may be so powerful that it always works, but if it fails and insomnia occurs it can easily become a sleepless ritual rather than a sleep one. Always bear in mind that normally your body automatically decides how much sleep you need and will make adjustments accordingly. So if one night you have had a long sleep and a lie-in the next morning, you will probably feel wide awake in the evening.

If you still feel fully alert at the time you would normally retire to bed there is no point in trying to go to sleep. Leave it until you feel tired and make the most of your extra waking time. On the other hand if you have had too little sleep you are likely to feel sleepy the next day. When you feel very drowsy, for example in your lunch hour after a heavy meal, it is sensible to have a quick catnap.

This may only last a few minutes but the sleep you get is valuable, and will protect you from irritability, headaches and the inefficiency that follows insomnia. The one exception to this rule is a cat-nap late in the evening just before going to bed. If this is taken too close to your normal sleeping time you are likely to be less sleepy when you go to bed and to have difficulty in getting off to sleep.

Remember that taking your sleep in one session of eight hours is merely a social convenience. Sleep is split up into two periods in many hot countries, one following the midday meal during the hottest hours of the day (the siesta), and the other late at night. By having an afternoon sleep you can stay up much later in the evening and need much less sleep at night. Older people tend to return to the sleep pattern of youth (the second childhood) and naturally prefer to sleep two or three times in the twenty-four-hour day. This pattern of sleep should be respected and not regarded as odd.

Boredom is an excellent assistant to sleep. You will probably recognize it as a problem during the day when you should be awake and alert. The long-distance driver, the airline pilot, the machinery supervisor, and the student swotting for exams all recognize the risk and the danger of falling asleep when working. The –insomniac ought to use boredom positively as an aid to sleep. As we noted earlier, constant change is needed to stay awake, and lack of change, or repetition, tends to make you drowsy. This is why those jobs which require regular concentration and yet involve little change are the most likely to make you sleepy. Driving in the narrow streets of a town is less likely to make you sleepy than driving on a motorway or freeway. When there are multiple pile-ups on motorways in bad weather conditions you read of 'motorway madness', but it is largely motorway boredom that is responsible. You become mesmerized by the car in front, your speed and engine sound stays constant and you stop thinking. You are quite ill equipped to deal with an emergency if one arises.

Anything which has a regular rhythm is likely to lead to boredom and sleepiness. This is best seen from the baby in a cradle, who can be transformed from a screaming, rigid mass into a peaceful, angelic figure in just a few minutes by the regular rocking movements. All the best lullabies have a simple regular rhythm which has the same effect. Many adults sleep better when on board ship, when the regular swell of the sea has the same rocking, sleepy quality. Of course in rough seas the rocking can become rather more violent and your sleep may be overtaken by seasickness. One insomniac I know only sleeps well when on board ship and has seriously considered converting his bed to a rocking one. Unfortunately his wife did not agree as she suspected that her job would be to rock it until he went to sleep. Some people think that the ideal rhythm for sleep is one that is the same as that of your heart-beat. Certainly rhythms that are a great deal faster or slower than the average heart-beat of 70 a minute are not so likely to make you sleepy.

One useful way of making yourself bored when you go to bed is to read a book. Clearly you have to choose the right book, as one in which you become absorbed will delay the onset of sleep. The most valuable bed-time book for the insomniac is one which starts well and arouses your interest immediately, but then slowly tails off so that you continue reading while only half concentrating. Many find detective stories suitable. All the important action comes in the first chapter and afterwards there is the tedious job of collecting evidence and following clues. Of course some people are such 'who-done-it' addicts that they have to read on to the end no matter how poor the book is, and they will have to choose a different kind of book to get off to sleep. It is also better to choose a small paperback than a heavy hardback book. The small one is easier to hold and is less likely to wake you up as it falls on your chest, the bed or the floor when you drop off to sleep. The size of print in a paperback is smaller and reading it can also make you feel more sleepy than when the print is large and bold.

What you eat also decides how you sleep and in recent years there has been much research on the foods that can cause insomnia and help sleep. Of course, it has been known for many years that good food and drink makes you feel sleepy. It has been said that the best tranquillizer in the world is a good square meal. But, like tranquillizers, good square meals are often habit-forming and although fat people have much less problem with sleeping than their skinny cousins, they are liable to suffer from many diseases which are more harmful than insomnia. The reason why people feel sleepier after eating is that the part of their nervous system that stimulates digestion is also the part that stimulates sleep. Your digestion is most active when you are asleep or resting and in general terms the more you eat the sleepier you will get.

Some drinks are also said to help sleep. You will have all seen advertisements for bedtime malted drinks, claiming that they promote sound, relaxed sleep. Advertisements often exaggerate, but this claim has been shown to be true for Horlicks and Ovaltine and probably applies to the others as well. Tea and coffee, on the other hand, contain caffeine, which is a stimulant. This prevents sleep and the insomniac is well advised to avoid these drinks completely in the three hours before bedtime.

Drinking a large volume of fluid may also affect sleeping.

We shall be talking about alcohol and sleep in a later chapter, but drinking large quantities of any liquid before going to bed is likely to interfere with sleep. Water does not need to be digested and so the part of your nervous
system concerned with relaxation and sleeping is not stimulated, although you may feel uncomfortably full.
And although your kidneys slow down during sleep they still have to get rid of excess fluid, so you are likely to be woken up several times in the night to pass water. This may not affect sleep much in the sound sleeper, but for the insomniac it is likely to prolong the waking hours.

Our last aid to sound sleeping is familiarity, which is closely bound up with security. The more used you are to a place, the better you will tend to sleep in it. If you have to sleep in a strange bed in a new house you will tend to sleep better if you have familiar articles with you. These may be your nightclothes, your alarm clock, or, of course, your sleeping partner. The best example of a familiar thing helping sleep is the favorite toy of a small child, the usually ragged and worn but much loved teddy bear or similar animal. In very young children it is often a piece of cloth or blanket. Whenever the child stays away from home with relatives or friends, or on holiday, the toy has to come with them, and woe betide the parents who forget to bring it. The fretful child refuses to go to sleep, cries over and over again for the single thing that will stop the tears, and no substitute will do. The toy is a symbol of security and continuity, it tells the child that although many things in the world can change, at least one will remain the same.

As adults we like to feel that we have got beyond this stage of development, but sleep brings out many of our most primitive wishes and needs. Many fully grown people still need these security symbols, although if they remain in the form of a cuddly bear, elephant or dolly their owners will do their best to hide it from others. If you are a parent and have a child of any age who still needs a toy like this, please respect this need and try not to make fun of him or her about it.

If the familiar things around us become associated with sleep, then all is well. For the chronic insomniac it is a different matter. If you have lain awake in your bedroom for hours, month after month or year after year, every feature becomes implanted in your memory. The ticking clock, the creaking left front leg of your bed, the pane of glass in the window that rattles with the slightest breeze, the bookcase and picture in the far corner that looks like a ghostly figure in the darkness. All these familiar sights and sounds become associated with not sleeping and therefore become unpleasant. For this desperate state of affairs desperate measures are needed. You may need to try one of the treatments described in the next two chapters, but beforehand you might try changing all these familiar features first. Try going to a different bedroom, or move the bedroom furniture around. You may also need to alter a great number of other habits that in most people are linked to sleep but in you have only led to insomnia. You might give up the hot shower you always have before going to bed, stop the familiar grandfather clock that cheerfully chimes every quarter of an hour and tells you how long you have been awake, or abandon the hot toddy that your uncle swears is the best cure for insomnia but which only gives you a headache the next morning.

Two other familiar things associated with good sleep in most people are also worth mentioning, darkness and silence. It is usually much easier to sleep at night than during the day, as shift workers often find out to their cost. Darkness is more restful to the eyes, and if you have to sleep during the day it is sometimes helpful to wear eye shades to cut down the light. Your eyelids are fairly good at cutting out light but you will notice that even if you shut your eyes in a bright light you are still aware of the light shining and causing your eyes to ache. The prevention of sleep by shining an intensely bright light is unfortunately only too well known by experts in the use of brain-washing, a process which involves sleep deprivation in its early stages.

Noise can also prevent sleep, although a regular noise can be soothing and soporific. It is sudden changes in noise that are the most upsetting for the insomniac, as they can wrench you away from sleep into complete wakefulness in a few seconds. Some people are very sensitive to noise, and nervous people in particular seem to be greatly affected. One of the things that troubles insomniacs when they are sleeping in unfamiliar surroundings is the difference in the background noise. When we go away from our homes we often go to places which are noisier, places like hotels, trains, holiday camps, the houses of relatives with young children, and so on. Even hospitals are affected and the lights are often on all night! It is other people who are responsible for most noise and if they would be more considerate it would be a great boon to the sleepless. The slogan 'noise almost always annoys' could be adopted with enthusiasm by all insomniacs.

If you are troubled by noise at night and nothing can be done to reduce it (please remember that shouting at the offender only makes more noise), then cut down the noise by wearing ear-plugs or muffs. Try not to block up the passage leading from your ears to the eardrum with cotton wool or other materials. If this is done regularly you can cause irritation and inflammation, or stimulate wax formation, which can block up your ears both night and day. Properly designed ear-plugs of the right size are comfortable and very effective in reducing noise. You can usually hear an alarm clock through them so do not let fear of oversleeping concern you too much. You are probably more easily woken than the average sleeper even when wearing ear-plugs.

When using these straightforward ways of helping your sleep, remember that no one requirement is absolutely essential for sleep. The statement 'I never sleep' cannot be true, nor can 'I never sleep at Aunt Ada's, the Grand Hotel, in that house with those awful children', or wherever it happens to be. You can sleep anywhere if you approach it in the right way. Sometimes insomnia is used as an excuse for not going somewhere or doing something which you would prefer to avoid. If this is the case, by all means claim insomnia as a white lie to avoid offence but be honest with yourself. If you are not, your phoney insomnia may become real insomnia and your suffering will really start.

Experiments have been done on people who live in the Antarctic or Arctic summers when the sun never sets. Here there is no means of telling what time of day it is from looking around. If sleep only took place in familiar surroundings and was decided by changes such as daylight disappearing, birdsong ceasing, the sight and feel of your soft, warm bed or the clock striking midnight, you would have no idea when to sleep and when to wake in the land of the midnight sun. In the experiments people have had their clocks and watches taken away and have no cues to help them to decide the time of day. This does not trouble them. Their sleep-waking rhythm takes over and they get all the sleep they need. Even if they are fooled into thinking that the day is longer or shorter than it really is (by giving them clocks that are too fast or too slow) their sleep rhythm continues more or less the same as before.

So even when you are asked to sleep in the strangest places you can adapt without much trouble, although the time it takes varies from person to person. You can help yourself to adapt more quickly by taking some of the elementary precautions we have mentioned, but even without them you will adapt in the end.

How to Control your Mind and Relax

We said earlier how important worrying was in causing insomnia. One of the reasons other animals do not seem to suffer from sleeplessness is that they do not worry, at least about sleep. They never give it a thought, and so their sleep is natural and uncomplicated. So insomniacs are repeatedly told: 'Try not to worry and everything will be all right'. Now this kind of advice infuriates people who cannot sleep. It implies that the reason they cannot go off to sleep is that they are deliberately worrying about something when they go to bed and if they would stop this silly habit all would be well. It also suggests that whether you worry or not is entirely under your control. The same sort of idea is implied in the remark: 'Just relax and you'll have no problem in getting to sleep'. All this kind of comment does is to make you feel even more tense with aggressive feelings towards the person who said it. Of course the presence of relaxation and the absence of worry will help sleep, but it is not achieved in the same way as turning a tap on or off when it suits you. What is even more annoying about this kind of superficial advice is that it is so often given with a smug, self-satisfied air which suggests that the speaker has indeed mastered this ability.

This is rarely true and he probably has just the same potential for insomnia as you.

But you should not give up trying to learn how to control your mind so that you can stop worrying, because it can be achieved. It usually requires help from others, which is why I have left it till the various forms of self-help have been tried first.

The knack you have to learn is the ability both to detach your mind so that it can, in effect, 'go blank', and also to concentrate it so that it can control the various changes going on in the body. This is asking a lot, because these are things that we normally never think of doing and have had no practice in attempting. In the East they have been practicing for centuries, and although we in the West were at first very skeptical of the value of these techniques, we are now much more humble. We still have a lot to learn.

One reason we were skeptical is that some of the ideas behind these techniques were, to say the least, far-fetched.

Take, for example, yoga. Yoga was originally one of the systems of Indian philosophy and parts of it have been changed over the centuries so that now it is thought of mainly as a system of mind control. But it is based on the idea that there is a divine female power at the bottom of the spine which can be connected by a system of 'wheels' to the chief center of power, which is male and is placed at the top of the brain. The aim of the person who practices yoga, called a yogi, is to unite the female and male powers so that complete salvation is achieved. This sort of explanation does not carry conviction to our Western ears, and the idea that the male is always superior to the female sounds like male chauvinism.

But of course the theories behind these techniques are less important than the question whether or not they work. Studies of yoga have shown that the mind has the power to control many parts of the body that normally we cannot influence. The yogi can make his heart beat extremely slowly and can also reduce the rate that his body uses energy so that he can survive for long periods without food or water. These feats are achieved by the professionals and no one is going to claim that you are going to be able to do the same. But even if you are only able to relax the tension in the muscles of your arms, legs and neck when you go to bed, this can make all the difference between staying awake or going to sleep.

Apart from yoga, there are other techniques with different names and origins but which share the same features, self-control of the mind and regulation of many of the body processes that go on automatically most of the time. Transcendental meditation is an extension from yoga which aims to improve your mental powers and thereby alter the whole function of your body. It has been shown to reduce high blood pressure and there is little doubt that, like yoga, it helps to relieve tension and will help insomnia if it is successfully achieved.

For insomniacs there are several simple yoga exercises which can help to relieve tension at night. Of course you can practice them at any time of day as well. The large number of yoga classes being set up and books and articles written on the subject show the tremendous interest that has been created by these techniques. I am not going to describe them in any detail but the following is a simple example. Lie flat on your back with your eyes closed, your feet stretched out and hands by your side. Concentrate on your breathing by taking slower and deeper breaths and also trying to breathe down into the bottom of your lungs rather than in the top of your chest. This should not be too difficult as we are all able to breathe with our chests or with our stomachs. Most of the time we do both but it is often unhealthy and inefficient. It may take a long time to unlearn the old ways of breathing but eventually you should learn this yoga breathing so your chest fills with air from the bottom of your lungs. As you do this you will find it is much easier to relax and you will feel the tension flowing from your muscles. At this stage you can focus on different muscles by concentrating and encouraging them to relax, feeling the muscles if you have any doubt whether you are succeeding. Then you feel your mind becoming freed from the restrictions of the body and can transport it to anywhere you wish, to a place where there is complete relaxation without any cares. All the time you continue your deep breathing and relaxation.

Your thinking should flow effortlessly otherwise you will find yourself building up tension again. Finally you can turn off the thought completely so your mind goes blank. No, you are not asleep, you have blown out the cobwebs of your mental cupboards and they are completely clean. This is a deep stage when your body rhythms will alter and set themselves at a lower level. You can keep this up for a few minutes or an hour or two before returning gradually to your normal state. When you return you will feel a different person and if tension has caused your insomnia you should now have no trouble in getting to sleep. Do not take this as a typical example of yoga, because I have left out much of the detailed instruction, but it should give you some idea of the technique.

I would advise you to try yoga or a similar technique first and see how it works for you. In most towns there are teaching classes for yoga, either during the day or in the evening, in which the basic techniques are taught, usually to groups of students. You can help by buying a book on the subject and continuing the exercises at home.

Once you have given it a fair trial you will probably find one of three results. The best, but usually least common, is that you master the main techniques and rapidly learn to control your insomnia. Once this happens you no longer worry about sleep and your problem is over.

Another way of reducing tension and anxiety is hypnosis. Although at first this usually involves the services of a hypnotist, if successful it can eventually be used alone and is then called auto-hypnosis. When people talk about hypnosis they often think of it as a technique of mind control. For the insomniac it appears to have all the attraction of yoga and none of its disadvantages. Instead of having to learn all these difficult ways of training your mind and body, you place yourself in the hands of an expert who will do it for you. Is hypnosis, therefore, the short cut to full relaxation and will it work if self-training has failed?

For most people the answer is no. Hypnosis can be useful, but not usually when other ways of trying to get to sleep have failed. This may disappoint you, particularly as a hypnotized person appears to be in a deep sleep after only a few minutes of treatment. It appears to be an almost instant cure for insomnia, so why is it not more widely

Or you may find that sometimes you can do everything right and are sure you have mastered the technique, only to find the next day you cannot make any progress at all.

Perhaps you cannot achieve full control because you are not picking up the cues your body is giving you, in which you are made very suggestible to the hypnotist, so that you will believe things he tells you which you would never believe in your normal state. For example you can be told that your right arm is completely numb and that you can no longer feel anything. In a hypnotic state you will believe this and will show no reaction if your right arm is prodded hard with a needle. But you will feel pain and draw your arm away sharply if your left arm is prodded with the needle in the same way. Good, you may say, put me into the same hypnotic trance and tell me I am asleep. This can be done, but you will not be really asleep. You will accept the suggestion that you are asleep but of course you are not, just in the same way that the hypnotized person told he has a numb right arm believes it to be true even though sensation in it is quite normal.

Brain waves have been measured in hypnotized people and are no different from the brain waves when they are awake, except in the deepest trances (which are difficult to achieve), when the waves are similar to those of light sleep.

When hypnosis is used to treat insomnia an indirect approach is used. The emphasis is put on relaxation and lessening anxiety when in the hypnotic trance. This can be done under light hypnosis and does not differ very much from the relaxation training we shall discuss later. The difficult thing is to transfer the value of this treatment from the hypno-therapist's consulting room to your own bedroom. When lying awake at night you cannot call on him for help and if you telephone him he will not be pleased. Some therapists may allow their voices to be taped when they are putting someone under hypnosis and although the tape-recorded voice without the person behind it is not so good as the real thing, it may often be of value.

There is another way of using hypnosis to treat insomnia.

You may have seen hypnosis practiced on the stage and marveled how quickly the hypnotist can put a volunteer from the audience into a deep trance just by saying a few words or merely by snapping his fingers. In these situations the 'volunteer' is already known to the hypnotist and has been hypnotized by him before. The reason he falls into a trance so quickly is because he has been given a post-hypnotic suggestion. This is a clever way of using the first hypnotic trance to make later trances much easier to achieve. What happens is that when the 'volunteer' is hypnotized for the first time by the hypnotist he is told during the trance that after he has recovered he will again return to the same trance whenever the hypnotist reacts in a certain way. This may involve saying a certain word or words, doing something such as jangling keys, snapping fingers, scratching the chin or a similar action which will mean nothing to a general audience. The hypnotist then tells the person that he will not be able to remember any of the things said to him during the trance.

He could also suggest that on recovery the person will also not be able to remember ever seeing the hypnotist before but will volunteer when the hypnotist appears on stage and asks for help with an experiment. Our poor subject is duly unaware of all this when he goes into the audience, volunteers as predicted and appears on stage. When the hypnotist carries out the post-hypnotic suggestion the audience do not think twice about it, but the pre-hypnotized volunteer recognizes it as a signal to which he responds by sinking into a deep trance. Whereas the first trance may take half an hour to achieve, the second happens in a few seconds.

In treating insomnia you can be put into a trance at your first hypno-therapy session and given a post-hypnotic suggestion that you will feel extremely relaxed, contented and sleepy whenever you hear a particular signal. This can be in a tape-recorded message to be played at your bedside, or the sound of your alarm clock being wound up at night. Care has to be taken not to make the signal one that could be heard or seen at other times of the day.

For example, an obvious post-hypnotic suggestion is that you should feel sleepy when your wife or husband says 'good-night' when you go to bed. But if you are out having dinner with friends in the evening and your host bids you good-night in a similar voice you are liable to fall asleep when driving home! Apart from this disadvantage there is a tendency for the post-hypnotic suggestion to be less effective the more often it is used, so you will probably need to have 'booster' visits to the hypnotist to keep up its strength.

Hypnosis can therefore be of value and live up to its name by treating insomnia, but it is not an easy task.

Many people do not reach the fairly deep trance level necessary to make good post-hypnotic suggestions and so the method is limited. You also need to remind yourself that whatever is achieved under hypnosis can be done by you alone. Hypnosis cannot make people what they are not, it merely brings into use powers that you did not know you had. If you, as well as a hypnotist, can draw on these powers when you need them it will give you greater confidence in controlling your insomnia, as well as saving you a great deal of money.

Another thing to realize is that the techniques of hypnosis can be learnt fairly easily and do not require a long period of specialized training. Most hypno-therapists do not have any formal qualifications and learn their skills quickly. Although they can claim with some justification that they have been shunned by the medical and the other caring professions and are not taken seriously enough, the fact is that the knowledge required to put someone into a hypnotic trance is small. If you practice hypnosis for a living you have to know more, chiefly about the types of disorder you can treat and which forms of hypnosis are most useful, and about its dangers. But if you suffer from insomnia and only wish to treat yourself, you may find self-hypnosis, also called auto-hypnosis, useful. This involves the two main parts of hypnosis, relaxation to the state of a light trance and the giving of suggestions to yourself while in this state. Obviously the insomniac will

give himself suggestions of drowsiness and sleepiness which should then lead to the onset of natural sleep. Again I emphasize that it is not a good idea to give yourself the suggestion that you are asleep because you may remain in a funny half-awake half-asleep state for a long time.

You are not really asleep but you may have convinced yourself you are. Natural sleep may take over but is more likely to do so only if you have suggested to yourself that you are drowsy.

All this may sound a little ridiculous. The idea of suggesting things to yourself in a state when you are likely to believe them must sound odd to the hard-headed insomniac. Never mind, perhaps we should put it to the test. Try the following exercise when you are lying in bed trying to get to sleep, or possibly in a warm, comfortable chair if you do not like reading flat on your back. The words in brackets tell you the things you should try to do and the other words should be repeated to yourself but not spoken out loud.

'I am going to feel completely relaxed and sleepy in a few minutes. It will only take a few minutes if I pay careful attention to the words I am reading and think of nothing else. I am listening to nothing else, nothing else at all. I am concentrating on these words, just these words. (Hold the book about six inches away from your eyes and look closely at every word.) As I look at these words I am thinking about nothing, nothing but the words. The words are helping me to feel relaxed but some of my muscles are still tense. My legs and arms are still tense but as I read these words I find my left leg is getting relaxed (move your left leg to a different position) and the tension is flowing away. And now my right leg is not so tense (move your right leg to a different position) and both legs are feeling more and more comfortable. And as they feel more comfortable they feel warmer. 1 can feel the warmth going into my legs and as it goes into my legs I feel my arms losing their tension (move your arms to a different position) and becoming more and more relaxed. The warmth is now travelling up my body and into my arms and I am feeling more and more comfortable. And now my whole body feels warm and relaxed and 1 find myself sinking into complete relaxation. And as I am getting more relaxed 1 find myself breathing slowly and deeply (take one deep breath), and with each breath I am getting more and more relaxed, breathing slowly and deeply and feeling more comfortable with each breath, till I am completely relaxed. And now 1 feel so relaxed my eyes are getting tired and I am finding it more difficult to read the words as 1 am feeling so drowsy and relaxed (close your eyes and open them slowly). My eyes feel so heavy 1 am finding it difficult to keep them open and I feel so relaxed I feel I must close my eyes. 1 am still looking at the words but I am feeling drowsy and relaxed, breathing deeply, so drowsy and relaxed, more and more comfortable, completely relaxed and comfortable, warm and relaxed, relaxed all over, completely relaxed' (close eyes).

If you have been reading this slowly and carefully, and concentrating on each of the words, you will have found that you are now a little sleepier than you were before, even if you have not been trying to get to sleep. The reason for this is fairly simple. I have used some of the techniques used by hypnotists to increase suggestibility.

Once this has happened, the further you read, the greater the effect of the instructions. So the last sentence has a much greater effect on you than very similar words written five sentences earlier. There is nothing particularly mysterious about the instructions and you may already have guessed why they have helped you to feel more relaxed from what I have already written about hypnosis.

If you have not, then do not be troubled. This simple beginning to auto-hypnosis will probably be all the more effective for you in fighting insomnia, so I will not explain further.

By repeating instructions like this over and over they will be remembered so you will not need to take the book to bed with you. You can also add instructions which are special to you, memories of your pre-sleep feelings which may be unique. Some feel detached from themselves in this state, or are completely still, unable to move even the smallest muscle, or have the experience of a rocking up and- down motion. Move on to these instructions when you have closed your eyes and you will find they help a great deal. When following these instructions without the book try and focus on a point six inches above your nose, or if you find this difficult, on the tip of your nose itself.

I would advise only using the full technique when you are trying to get to sleep, and not at other times when you feel tense. You will probably have picked up enough to help you combat extreme tension if you suffer from this, but it may also require some practical instruction in the art of relaxation. Relaxation classes are held in many evening institutes and are often combined with yoga. You will usually take part in these classes in groups and any difficulties you have in getting relaxed can be overcome by practice and by talking with your instructor and other pupils.

Throughout this chapter you will have noticed that the same principles have come up time and time again: the training of your mind to focus on one thing to the exclusion of all others, the ability to change the workings of your body, and the art of relaxation. From the point of view of the insomniac, yoga, transcendental meditation, zen and similar techniques, hypnosis and relaxation training all involve these principles with different degrees of emphasis. The theories behind them could not be more different but in practice they share a great deal. There is one other important ingredient, belief. If you believe when you are trying these ways of solving insomnia that they are going to work, they are more likely to do so. I realize it is asking a lot of a chronic insomniac to believe that some new treatment is going to work when everything else has failed. He stopped believing a long time ago and is skeptical of any new approach. Lack of belief may be a barrier to progress with these treatments but not an absolute one. Keep working at them and once you have achieved a little, belief in your abilities will grow and more will follow. Once this has happened you will be amazed at the powers that are immediately available to you.

There are some words of warning which apply most to the insomniacs who find these forms of help the best way of 'curing' their insomnia. I put 'curing' in inverted commas because by sleeping well again you have not necessarily cured yourself. If your insomnia is caused by worry about your marriage, the absence of any meaning in your life, or the many unpaid bills you cannot meet because of debt, then the mere fact of sleeping well again is not going to help in the long run. In these cases your insomnia is drawing attention to a problem about which you must do something more than try and get a good night's sleep. So before you sign up for your yoga class or practice your meditation, ask yourself whether your insomnia might be a warning signal about something that is wrong in your life. You may decide that there is no real cause for you not sleeping or you may pick on the wrong cause. The real cause may stay buried for a long time before you uncover it. So if your insomnia seems to have no end you should keep asking yourself whether there is something else which might be behind it, something which you have ignored, forgotten, or dismissed as unimportant.

If you find that auto-hypnosis helps to get you off to sleep but has to be gone through night after night, and that insomnia always comes back if you do not keep your self-treatment going, then one of these hidden causes is likely.

The second warning concerns the dangers of the types of treatment involving mind and body control. I mentioned earlier that professional hypnotists have to be trained and that a great part of their training is concerned with the limits and dangers of hypnosis. Now if you find that hypnosis, or any of the other treatments we have talked about, is effective in helping you 10 relax and sleep, you might find it hard to accept that it could have any dangers in your case. But it does. If you stop and think what happens in these treatments you will see that they are all inward-looking. They teach you a lot about yourself and your powers and therein lies their value. But there is another side to the coin. Because they are inward-looking they carry the danger of making you so bound up in yourself that nothing else seems to matter. You, your feelings, body's reactions and mental powers become your real world, and the hurly-burly of the world outside, where your mind and body have no control, becomes a fantasy.

Of course, it is really you who are living in a fantasy world. Inner peace and tranquility may feel nice but they will not pay the milkman or cook the dinner.

So by all means learn these techniques to improve your sleep and your mental and bodily health, but do not overindulge them. Once you start practicing them for their pleasurable feelings alone you are running into danger.

Remind yourself that all the Eastern treatments are founded on the concept of balance. Health is only obtained when positive and negative qualities (the yin and yang of Chinese philosophy) are exactly equal. Weigh up the positive and negative parts of the treatments you try and make sure that balance is maintained.

Pills, Medicines and Sleep

No, this chapter is not just about sleeping pills. We live in a tablet-taking, medicine-guzzling society in which pills and potions are prescribed for every kind of ailment, as well as for sleep. The reason I am including other medicines here is that many of them alter your sleeping habits, either because they are stimulants and wake you up, or are sedatives which make you feel drowsy. It would be quite wrong to leave them out of a book on insomnia as they may have a great deal to do with not sleeping.

But first let us deal with sleeping pills and medicines, which are called hypnotics by doctors. Do you take sleeping pills now or have you ever taken them in the past?

If you have, you will probably feel guilty about admitting it, the same sort of guilt you might feel about not being able to control your drinking, or about that affair you had with that older woman when you were not quite eighteen.

Why do you feel guilty? If someone asked you if you had ever taken an aspirin before you would not mind admitting it. You might even tell the questioner how many aspirins you consume regularly to impress on them how much pain you have had. But with sleeping pills you reply sheepishly that you feel guilty because taking these tablets suggests that you have a kind of weakness. If only you had the strength to cope with insomnia or learn healthier ways of controlling it you would be a more respectable person.

But I can argue back that taking an aspirin is also a sign of weakness if you look at it in the same way. If you whether you would do this if an aspirin or a similar painkilling tablet was at hand. You would take the tablet and think nothing more about it. Another reason for feeling guilty about taking sleeping pills is that they 'affect the mind'. Taking a tablet for heart or kidney trouble is quite all right, but taking one for the mind is another matter.

This is the 'Mysterious Black Box' argument. We know how the heart and kidneys work but the mind is a mystery, therefore we should not tamper with it in case something goes badly wrong. But, I will counter, the aspirin you take for your toothache also acts on your mind. When the aspirin takes away the pain the toothache is still there; the aspirin has only altered the pain threshold in your brain so you do not feel the ache in your jaw. The way in which aspirin works is still a mystery after a hundred years of use so this argument does not hold up either.

The reasons for feeling guilty therefore all seem a bit silly. If they apply to sleeping pills they should apply to pain-killers and a large number of other tablets. But there are other reasons which are more sensible and should make you look at sleeping pills with caution. The main one is that many of them are habit forming. As we shall see later there are many differences between them and you are more likely to get hooked on some than others. A second reason may be connected with the first: the taking of sleeping pills is increasing so fast that at the present rate of progress it looks as though most people will be taking them, at least occasionally, by the end of this century. To give you some idea of this rate of increase, the number of prescriptions for sleeping pills and tranquillizers today in England and Wales is nearly three times as many as twenty years ago. In just one year there are forty-six million prescriptions for these pills, that is an average of nearly one prescription for every man, woman and child.

This increase is recent and before twenty years ago you would not have felt so guilty about taking sleeping tablets. have toothache you are stronger, in the mental sense, if you do not take an aspirin for it. You can sit there heroically enduring your pain without a murmur. But I doubt People have been taking sleeping medicines for years. The Chinese have records going back two thousand years of the use of opium for sleeping, and although there must have been many who were addicted to opium for sleep there were few who were really bothered by this. Only a hundred years ago Sigmund Freud said that another highly addictive drug, cocaine, was a marvelous cure for sleeping problems as well as other nervous complaints.

At the time he had only just discovered cocaine and no one knew how dangerous it was. So modern doctors who prescribe sleeping pills are now sadder and wiser men; they do not use words like 'cure' when they talk about pills for insomnia and they often talk about 'dependence', a mild form of addiction which can be a problem with so many sleeping tablets.

If you find you cannot stop taking your particular sleeping tablet it is not really you who should be feeling guilty, but the doctors who prescribed them for you in the first place, and the drug companies who make and sell the tablets. But those who take the odd sleeping tablet from time to time or have taken a short course in the past should have no feelings of guilt, and nor should anyone else.

And as we shall see, the sleeping tablets of today are a great deal safer and better than the ones of only fifteen years ago. Do sleeping tablets work? Can two million people be wrong when they take their magic capsule to get them off to sleep? Yes, they can be wrong, because even if taking a tablet leads to sleep it could be nothing to do with the tablet. In the last chapter we found that if you believe that yoga and similar techniques will help your insomnia they will be more likely to work. The same applies to sleeping tablets. If you believe your tablet will get you off to sleep you will no longer worry about staying awake and natural sleep will follow. I say 'natural sleep' because even if the capsule does have a knockout effect it takes at least half an hour to get absorbed into your body, and if you go to sleep after ten minutes it cannot be due to the actual drug inside the capsule. The belief that a treatment will work will often make it work even if it is completely useless.

This is often called 'the placebo effect'. 'Placebo' is a Latin word meaning 'I will please', and indeed it does please. The big advantage of taking a completely useless treatment that appears to work is that it cannot have any real dangers. It is a sad fact that any treatment that is good for insomnia carries with it at least one or two dangers, but the placebo is harmless. But why bother with real sleeping tablets at all if the placebo or dummy tablet is so good? Alas, this powerful placebo effect does not last more than a few days and many people do not notice it at all.

You are more likely to notice the effect the more you trust in the treatment. The skeptical insomniac who takes the view that nothing will cure his sleeplessness apart from a hard blow from a hammer on his head each night (a treatment which he does not actually take because of possible side effects) is not going to be fooled by a dummy tablet.

So doctors nowadays rarely use placebo tablets except for special reasons.

Although many of the sleeping medicines of years ago were really placebos, fooling both the doctors and their patients when they worked, the sleeping tablet you get when you go to the chemist with a prescription is the real thing. It has been developed from many years of research and has been proved to be a help in getting to sleep. This does not mean that it will necessarily work for you, it tells us that most people with insomnia will sleep better after taking the tablet than if, for example, they had taken a dummy pill.

If you have never taken a sleeping pill you may like to know what happens. As the tablet or capsule takes some time to be absorbed into the body you will probably notice nothing for at least twenty minutes. If you find something dramatic happens in only a few minutes our friend the placebo effect is playing a game with you. After about half an hour you begin to feel sleepy. This feeling is often like natural drowsiness but sometimes comes on so rapidly you may find it hard to stay awake. You will normally go to sleep within another half-hour and, if all goes well, you will stay asleep till morning. The stages of sleep that we mentioned in the second chapter are gone through in cycles throughout the night, apart from one important difference. With many sleeping tablets there is less time spent in rapid eye movement (REM) sleep than normal, and sometimes REM sleep may disappear altogether. This means that you spend less time dreaming and your sleep cannot be described as natural sleep. The deeper stages of sleep may also be less frequent with sleeping tablets.

It is not certain whether this loss of REM sleep does any harm but it is unlikely to do any good. What is known is that when you finish a course of sleeping tablets that reduce REM sleep, for about six weeks afterwards you will have more REM sleep and will also dream more. We come back again to the balancing mechanisms in the body. In just the same way as you make up lost ordinary sleep by sleeping longer, you make up lost REM sleep by dreaming longer. All this suggests that REM sleep is important and that you are depriving yourself in some way if you take sleeping tablets for too long.

When you wake up in the morning after a sleeping tablet you are unlikely to feel completely fit and ready to go. Your alarm clock will probably take a little longer to wake you and you will feel tired and sluggish. You roll out of bed bleary-eyed and it seems to take ages before you wake up completely. Even when you are properly awake you do not feel quite right; your head feels muzzy, you cannot concentrate properly and you may have difficulty getting your balance. If you have never taken a sleeping tablet before you will probably still recognize the feeling.

It is the feeling of 'the morning after the night before', or hangover. Not surprisingly, therefore, these effects of sleeping pills are called hangover effects and all medicines taken for sleep can have these effects, although they are much commoner with some than others. At this point we should also remind ourselves that alcohol has been used for years as a sleeping medicine so hangover is a good word to describe these effects. As well as noticing these unpleasant feelings other people will also notice that you are not as quick on the uptake as normal. So if you are driving to work and have to stop suddenly in an emergency
you will react less quickly and this can make all the difference between avoiding an accident and having one.

The hangover effects usually last for a few hours but can often be found much later in the day. There is no such thing as the ideal sleeping pill that sends you off to sleep immediately and allows you to wake completely refreshed in the morning without any after-effects. If everybody knew this many people would be less happy about starting them in the first place. After reading about the problems you can have with them you may think it curious that they are prescribed at all. But you have to remember that insomnia also creates unpleasant feelings-irritability, poor concentration, drowsiness and headaches-and if you have a good night's sleep with a sleeping pill you will probably feel better in the morning than if you have been awake half the night. Often the delayed reactions that follow taking a sleeping pill are not noticed. You feel better after a good night's sleep, get into your car and drive recklessly into town, completely unaware that you are a danger on the road. If you are involved in an accident and it becomes known that you have been taking sleeping pills this is likely to count against you.

Up to now we have been talking about sleeping pills in general, but there are over forty different types of sleeping medicine that you may be prescribed, and it is helpful to know some of the differences between them.

Until a few years ago the commonest sleeping tablets were the barbiturates. They certainly help you to get off to sleep but not in the right way. Instead of just working on the part of your brain that is concerned with sleep they interfere with all your mental processes. It is like asking for an ear-plug to cut down noise and having a blanket thrown over your head and pulled tight. The noise gets less, but you cannot see or smell either. Barbiturates dull the brain and the hangover effects you get on waking are much worse than with most other kinds of sleeping tablet.

But this is not their worst problem. That is addiction. It is right to use the word 'addiction' with barbiturates, because the true addict gets so used to having a drug inside his system that he cannot do without it. If the drug is suddenly stopped he suffers from severe and sometimes dangerous reactions called withdrawal symptoms. The only way he knows of taking away these nasty feelings is to take more of the drug, so he is well and truly hooked.

One type of withdrawal reaction you may have read about or come across before is delirium tremens, or D.T.s, as it is so often called. This only happens in people who are addicted to alcohol; people who have taken large quantities of alcohol (in any form) for months and years, and then suddenly stop. At first they feel uneasy and nervous, and later they become terrified, shake all over and imagine they see rats, spiders or other frightening animals or shapes coming towards them. The often quoted stories of seeing pink elephants dancing in the air are rarely true; the visions (correctly called hallucinations) are much more frightening than that. These feelings may go on for several days and treatment in hospital is usually needed. Once he has got over this state the addict will remain well, provided he does not return to drinking too much alcohol again, and many advise that complete abstinence is the only answer.

If you are an insomniac you may think this kind of problem could never happen with you because you are strong enough to control it. This is dangerous talk, for you often drift into addiction gradually; by the time you realize what has happened it is too late, and your willpower cannot rescue you on its own. Alcohol is very similar to the barbiturates in its effects on the brain, yet many who would never think of taking sleeping pills take it regularly at night to help with insomnia. The danger signals are the same with both alcohol and barbiturates.

You first find that instead of taking the drink or the pill occasionally you take it regularly every night. You may even convince yourself that you do not really need it and are only taking it as an insurance policy in case of trouble.

The next stage is that you increase the number of tablets or the amount you drink each night. This can take place very gradually, so gradually that you are often unaware of it yourself. The reason you take more is that your body has got used to the drug-yes, alcohol is a drug too-and more is needed to produce the same effect. If you do not recognize the problem at this point you are on the slippery slope to real addiction. Before long the only time you feel well is when you have taken the drug, but larger and larger amounts are needed to keep this feeling of wellbeing.

The main purpose of life becomes the search for more supplies of the drug, if necessary through illegal means. Your job, your family, your property and your principles all take second place to the drug need and you become a mockery of your former self.

You have probably all heard of the 'skid row' alcoholic, a pathetic figure who is reduced to drinking methylated spirits, hair lacquer, and surgical spirit to keep his alcohol level up, who leaves or is left by his family and wanders the streets from one doss house to another. These people were not always like this; most were ordinary members of the community, part of the respectable society that now looks on them with pity or scorn. The same can happen with the barbiturate addict, although such addicts are less common now that barbiturates are not so often prescribed.

There are still skid row barbiturate addicts, usually younger than their alcoholic counterparts, but equally pathetic. As well as swallowing barbiturates in the usual way they crush the tablets, mix them with water and inject them into their veins. They are 'main-liners', like many heroin and opium addicts, and indeed often move on to taking these other dangerous drugs as well. If they cannot get hold of their drugs they may have a similar reaction to the alcohol addict on withdrawal, a barbiturate equivalent of delirium tremens in which hallucinations, shaking and fits can all happen.

If you are taking barbiturates for insomnia you should therefore think seriously about stopping them and replacing them with a safer type of sleeping pill. If you do not, your doctor will probably take the decision on your behalf before long. At the same time you should not presume that everyone who takes a barbiturate regularly is an addict. There are some who take them for years and who rarely increase the dose. But they are running the risk of becoming addicted each time they have to increase the dose for any reason. They are walking a tightrope and must always be on their guard. The longer you take a barbiturate

the more difficult it is to stop and so the sooner you kick the habit the better. Any withdrawal symptoms you have on stopping will be greater if you delay, and your doctor has ways of reducing these symptoms so that they are much less troubling.

One or two barbiturates are taken for good medical reasons and do not carry the same risks. The main one is phenobarbitone (Luminal) which is taken for epilepsy and very occasionally for feelings of anxiety. This does not have the same dangers as other barbiturates and can be taken for a long time without danger.

How do you know if the sleeping pill you are prescribed, or have been taking, is a barbiturate? There are always two names for any drug, the proper approved name of the tablet which is the same throughout the world, and a trade name which varies from one drug company to another and from country to country. As a general guide, if the approved name of the drug ends in 'barbitone' it is a barbiturate. The trade names of the commonest barbiturates used for insomnia are Sodium Amytal, Seconal, Nembutal and Tuinal and if you are prescribed these at any time there is no harm in questioning the doctor about the need to take them. There are other sleeping pills which are less dangerous and just as effective. These named drugs are not the only barbiturates available and there are many other drugs that are combinations of barbiturates with other substances. Now you will seldom receive a prescription for any drug containing barbiturates but if in doubt ask your doctor or chemist. It is better to know

in advance of any problems.

There are even more dangers in taking barbiturates. Because they dampen down all parts of the brain they can be dangerous if you take more than the recommended dose. All parts of the brain go to sleep, including the centers that are responsible for your breathing and your circulation. If they stop working you die. This is why overdoses of barbiturates are often fatal. There are even cases on record when an overdose has been taken by accident.

Some people have the unwise habit of keeping their sleeping pills on their bedside cabinets. They take their normal one or two tablets at night when they go to bed but often still wake up in the early hours. They are not aware of what is going on when they wake up and in their drugged state they may forget they have taken their sleeping pills already. But finding themselves awake and seeing from their clock that it is the middle of the night they take some more sleeping pills. Later, when they are recovering in hospital from their overdose they cannot remember what

went wrong. They certainly had no intention of committing suicide but their automatic habit of reaching for the bottle of sleeping tablets almost cost them their lives.

The right place for all drugs is the medicine cabinet, locked away so no accidents like this can happen. Children will be protected too. A normal adult dose can be fatal for a baby. Another unfortunate cause of death when taking barbiturates is the harmful effect it has when taken with alcohol or any other drugs that act on the brain in the same way. After a night of moderately heavy drinking the normal dose of barbiturates can kill.

The barbiturate story is not a happy one and is a timely reminder for all who take sleeping pills. Although many of the other types of tablet are much less dangerous, they have many of the same unpleasant effects in miniature.

The group of tablets that is most often prescribed for sleep problems today contains some drugs that are so common that they have become household names. The trade names of the most familiar ones are Valium,

Librium, Mogadon and Dalmane. Their proper names often end in '-azepam', so Valium is diazepam, and Mogadon is nitrazepam. These tablets are now preferred to barbiturates in treating insomnia and are often used for treating anxiety as well. In fact Valium is at present the most commonly prescribed drug in the world. It is easy to see why a treatment for anxiety is also one for insomnia.

Anxiety and worry run together and lead to difficulty in relaxing and muscular tension. Once anxiety has been removed in someone who would otherwise be sleepy at the end of the day, then sleep will follow. The sleep following these tablets is more natural than that following barbiturates.

There is little effect on REM sleep and dreaming, and there is much less danger from overdose, almost none at all if they are taken without any other drug. The reason they are safer is that they only affect the part of brain concerned with anxiety and sleep, unlike the blanket effect
of the barbiturates.

You might think this is marvellous. Here is a tablet that switches off nervousness and tension at its source in the brain, and solves sleeplessness. But it is not as simple as that. These drugs also have their hangover effects, not as bad as the barbiturates, but still enough to spill over
 into the next day. They too affect your concentration and fine movements, so you drive less well and make more mistakes in skilled jobs. And there is also a problem with dependence, although it is very rare to get addiction as with the barbiturates. It used to be thought that you did not get dependent on these tablets, but after they had been used for several years more and more people found that they could not stop taking the tablets.

There may have been a perfectly good reason why they started on the tablets in the first plate, such as a major upset following a death in the family, but once the crisis was over the tablets were still needed. If you are in this position and have been taking a tablet such as Mogadon every night for over a year there could be several reasons why you cannot stop. The first, and the most unlikely, is that you have been an insomniac all your life and it is only since you have been taking the tablets regularly that you have slept well. Or you may have been a nervous person all your life and the hangover effects of your tablets are relaxing rather than unpleasant because they take the edge off your anxiety. More commonly you are afraid to stop them in case your insomnia returns and you prefer not to take the risk. It is also possible that you have stopped the tablet occasionally and found you could not sleep, so quickly started taking them again.

At this stage there are no obvious dangers in continuing the same tablets for as long as you wish. But the longer you continue them the more likely you are to get used to their effects and have to increase the amount you take.

With these tablets the increase is much more gradual than with the barbiturates and you are even less likely to notice it. You may think when there is a small increase that it is because you have put on some weight, or because you have had a few more worries recently, but in reality your body has got used to the tablet and is quietly but insistently asking for more. Only in a few people is there a rapid increase in the number of tablets taken, leading to addiction and a withdrawal syndrome when the tablets are stopped. This is very rare and only a handful of cases have been reported, although millions of people take these tablets every day. So with Librium, Mogadon and Valium you are not on the way to skid row if you find you cannot stop taking the tablets, but the longer you remain on them the more difficult it will be to break the habit. When you do stop you may have a few sleepless nights and some anxiety symptoms like headache, palpitations or irritability, but if you stick it out these will go, and the earlier you stop the tablets the less severe these feelings will be.

When you read of the massive increase in the number of prescriptions for sleeping pills you need to realize that most of the prescriptions are repeat ones. So although the number of people taking sleeping pills is increasing steadily, the number of prescriptions is increasing much more quickly, as so few are finishing their 'course of treatment'.

Most of the repeat tablet-takers can stop their course and should have the courage at least to try. It is not just a medical decision to be left to your doctor. What I find most troubling about the continuous consumption of pills like these is the effect it has on other members of the family. If you take a sleeping pill regularly there is a danger that you will be seen as ill, a handicapped member of the family that needs to be propped up by pills. You can then be ignored when important decisions need to be taken, or unnecessarily protected when there is some threat from outside. Gradually your independence is whittled away and if you are not careful you can lose your self-respect. You take on the role that others have prepared for you, start behaving as an invalid, and often turn to other pills when they are not needed. Before these attitudes have a chance to become established you should make a determined effort to stop the regular nightly pill.

Enlist the help of your doctor and the family and get them on your side. They would all like you to be free of tablets again and will be pleased to co-operate.

There are other sleeping pills and medicines that come in between the barbiturates and the Valium group. They include Welldorm, Tricloryl, Oblivon and Doriden. It is wise to think of the last two in the same way as barbiturates, because you can get an addiction syndrome with them. Again the first sign is an increase in the number of tablets that you appear to need, and you often take them during the day as well as at night. Welldorm and Tricloryl are based on a drug called chloral. It is a relatively safe medicine that is much older than most of the other tablets I have mentioned but it is not quite as powerful as some of them. Dissolved in syrup it is often used as a sleeping medicine for babies and very young children and is quite effective. It is interesting that young children are usually given sleeping medicines correctly. They are only given occasionally at times of difficulty like teething or with measles and similar childhood diseases. Their parents recognize the need to give the drugs temporarily to help over a difficult period. It is curious that the same people often cannot look after their own sleeping tablets in the same sensible way.

One last tablet which deserves a mention is meprobamate (Equanil). Sometime ago this was hailed as the wonder drug for anxiety and insomnia and under the name of Miltown it became the most frequently prescribed drug in the United States. It was said to be non-habit forming and completely free of addiction, and to 'relax the person for natural sleep'. We know now that it is fairly good at relaxing tense muscles but not particularly good as a sleeping tablet, will interfere with the different stages of sleep, and can be addictive in regular dosage.

So we continue to learn, slowly.

I hope the last few pages have shown that it is quite wrong to think that all sleeping pills are the same. Yet the ones I have described make up only about two-thirds of the medicines used for getting off to sleep. Many other tablets make you feel sleepy as a side-effect, and sometimes they are used mainly as sleeping tablets. Among these are sea-sickness pills. If you have ever taken any of these pills to stop yourself feeling sick on a boat or car journey you may have noticed that you felt drowsy afterwards and possibly went to sleep for a short time. The idea of taking these tablets is to prevent queasy sick feelings, and not to make you go to sleep, much as you may have thought otherwise. It so happens that all the tablets that help sea-sickness have these dozy effects, some more than others. When they are taken late at night they will have the same effect as a mild sleeping tablet, and in children are often used for this purpose. As a general rule any tablet that causes drowsiness can help sleep. This can be put to good use if you have to take other tablets for any reason. Many of the tablets used to control blood pressure, heart disease, skin rashes and pain can make you feel sleepy as well. Your doctor may even advise you to take some of these tablets late at night because of this.

In this way you can have a good night's sleep and be free of drowsiness the next day. An even larger proportion of the drugs used to treat mental illness have the same properties, and the time you take them can also be altered in the same way. Always ask medical advice before you decide to do this, because some medicines have to be taken at certain times, like insulin for diabetes, and it would be dangerous to change the times of taking these.

Many medicines have the opposite effect: they are stimulants, not sedatives. A stimulant can speed up the body and the brain, increasing anxiety and excitement, and this may prevent sleep. You cannot always tell which medicines are stimulants from your own reactions to them. Many think alcohol is a stimulant because it seems to pep you up and make life more interesting. In fact, as we discussed earlier, it is a sedative which is rather similar to the barbiturates. In small doses, barbiturates also make you feel excited and more active, in exactly the same way as alcohol, which is one of the reasons drug addicts like them so much. These changes take place with alcohol and barbiturates because in small doses they remove many of your inhibitions by 'sedating' higher mental influences. In short, you put your conscience to sleep before other parts of your brain. This is why people often behave quite differently after a few drinks from their normal highly controlled selves, and feel very ashamed about their behavior when they wake the next morning!

Many say the person you see under the influence of alcohol is the real person, warts and all, and the same person when sober is only presenting the part of himself that he wants the world to see.

False stimulants like alcohol and barbiturates can be identified easily, for when you take a large quantity you become very sleepy. With real stimulants you become more sleepless and excited. As we noted earlier, tea and coffee are real stimulants and it is unwise to take them too close to bedtime. Another stimulant drug, and an addictive one at that, is nicotine. Nicotine, of course, is found in cigarette and pipe tobacco, and if you are a smoker who has tried to give up the habit you will have some idea what addiction and withdrawal symptoms are like. The habit of smoking late at night is not advisable if you are an insomniac, as with each inhalation of smoke you are getting more tense and awake. The habit of smoking in bed has even less to commend it. Quite apart from keeping you awake, filling your bedroom with tar and smoke, poisoning the atmosphere and making you cough, it is also a fire risk. If you drop off to sleep when smoking--even stimulants will not keep you awake all night-you can easily set fire to your bedclothes, most of which are highly inflammable.

If you are addicted to smoking and cannot sleep I would advise giving up cigarettes before you add another addiction, sleeping pills, to your smoking.

Many stimulant drugs can be bought at a chemist's or drug store without a prescription, and as they may interfere with sleep you should be aware of them. The most common are medicines to help with breathing. Drops which dry up the nose when it is bunged up after a heavy cold, open up the breathing tubes in conditions like asthma, and control sinus infections, are almost all stimulants.

You can often be in a dilemma deciding whether you are more likely to stay awake because you cannot breathe comfortably or because you have taken a stimulant medicine.

The amount of stimulation depends on how much of the tablet gets into the bloodstream. If you use nose drops very little will be absorbed; more will be absorbed with aerosol sprays, and most when you take a tablet or suppository.

If you have to take tablets or treatments like these regularly and find you have difficulty in sleeping it might be helpful to discuss it with your doctor to see if some changes can be made. Some tablets that are used to treat migraine have stimulant properties as well. Caffeine, the important stimulant of both tea and coffee, is contained in them. Many slimming pills are also stimulants and can affect sleeping if taken too late in the evening. There are many other stimulants and it would be difficult to list them all, but if you are on the lookout for causes of your insomnia, do not forget other tablets, no matter for what reason you are taking them.

When stimulants are combined with sedatives some peculiar things can happen. One of the notorious combinations is Drinamyl, a combination of amphetamine with a barbiturate. Drinamyl used to be very popular because it appeared to be an almost instant reliever of depression and other unpleasant moods. It also reduced appetite and was fancied by slimmers, and generally made people livelier and more enthusiastic. Unfortunately these effects get out of control once the tablets are taken regularly. You rapidly get used to the pills, take more of them and are quickly addicted. The loss of appetite often gets out of control and you lose much more weight than you intend, and you find that the only way you can stay feeling happy is to keep on the tablets, as you suffer deep depression when they are withdrawn. To cap it all, you often have persistent insomnia, which does not trouble you at first but will if it lasts. Amphetamine itself is one of the 'soft' drugs much favoured by drug addicts.

The instant lift it gives is at first desired, then demanded, and finally becomes the main point of living. Addiction happens very quickly indeed and you can develop severe mental illness with delusions that you are being persecuted.

Insomnia is severe, but becomes the least of the addict's problems.

Amphetamines and similar drugs such as Drinamyl are now seldom prescribed and are banned in many places, but not long ago they were respectable drugs prescribed by respectable doctors who wished to do the best for their patients. The conventional medicines of today can become the banned drugs of tomorrow, because it is only when tablets have been used for many years that all their advantages and disadvantages are known. Eighteen years ago one of the most favored new sleeping tablets was thalidomide.

It was excellent at promoting sleep, did not seem to be habit-forming and had few hangover effects. It remains an excellent sleeping tablet but whatever benefit it gave to sleep was more than taken away by its other effects on the unborn baby. The tragedy of thalidomide is now well known to everyone, but most of all to the mothers who know that but for their insomnia in pregnancy their personal tragedy would never have taken place. Doctors are now extremely cautious about prescribing any tablets in the first few months of pregnancy. If you think you may be expecting a baby and have any sleep disturbance, then avoid taking tablets unless it is felt to be absolutely necessary.

After reading this chapter of errors and accidents you may be put off sleeping pills for life. If so, I shall be pleased, for it is a sound and healthy attitude. But if you find you do need them, you will want to know which tablets to take, how to take them and for how long? All sleeping pills have to be prescribed by doctors and obviously you will be guided by him to some extent in all these matters. This particularly applies to the choice of tablets. You must tell him if you have any allergies to pills as this may affect the choice, and the effects of any sleeping tablets you have had before may also be worth a mention. As we noted earlier, barbiturates should usually be avoided and if you are prescribed one of these do not be afraid to question it. There has been a recent campaign in the United Kingdom to discourage doctors from prescribing barbiturates. The campaign has not been organized by a pressure group but by the doctors themselves, so you are on good ground if you do voice your doubts. The other kinds of sleeping pill may all have a place in the treatment of insomnia.

You can have a much greater say in how you take your tablets. They can either be prescribed regularly every night or to be taken when required. There is seldom any need for a tablet to be taken regularly if it is taken for sleep alone. When you think about this it is fairly obvious.

The idea of a sleeping pill is to encourage sleep and if you are feeling naturally drowsy after a hard day's work it is pointless taking a sleeping pill. If natural sleep is likely, then give it a chance to work, instead of forcing an unnatural sleep on yourself. If your prescription says 'take one or two tablets as required', it usually means 'take no tablets or one or two as required'. You are the person who decides what is best on the basis of your own feelings. Similarly, if you are going to bed in an emotionally disturbed, excited state and there are good reasons for having a sound night's sleep, then it is reasonable to take the two tablets allowed. But remember not to go beyond the maximum allowed. If, of course, you are taking a tablet for another purpose and only take it at night rather than by day because it helps sleep, then you should take this regularly.

By keeping a close check on your feelings and only taking sleeping tablets when you need them, you are helping yourself in several ways. First, you are taking the smallest number of tablets necessary for good sleep and are interfering with normal sleep much less than if you take more tablets. Many other sleeping tablets apart from barbiturates interfere with REM sleep and dreaming, but only when they are taken in larger doses. Secondly, you are preventing a build-up of tablets in your system which can cause many problems. Many sleeping pills take a long time to be got rid of by the body and if they are taken regularly you gradually accumulate more of the tablets inside you.

You can guess what happens then. All the unpleasant hangover effects, muzzy feelings, difficulty in concentrating and slowness of reactions, spill over into the day so that you are in danger of becoming continuously tranquillized whether you want to be or not. Thirdly, and possibly most importantly, you are preventing yourself becoming dependent on the sleeping pill. There are two kinds of dependence: one which is found with drugs of addiction known as physical dependence, and a milder form which is called psychological dependence. In psychological dependence you are not really addicted but you feel you cannot do without something that you ought to be able to do without. That something may be a tablet, a pet, a habit such as gambling, or a food like cheesecake.

You do not need any of these things but when dependent on them you cannot break yourself of the need without a great deal of trouble. There have even been reports of people who are dependent on placebo tablets, dummy pills that contain nothing but chalk. So if you take sleeping tablets every night and find they work, you are tempted to go on taking them even if the original need to take them has disappeared long ago. Once you are in the habit you will almost certainly have difficulty in sleeping again when you stop the pills, just because you expect your insomnia to return. In any case you will go through a period of readjustment when sleeping will be temporarily disturbed if you have been on sleeping tablets regularly for a few weeks or more.

So if you use sleeping pills sensibly all these problems can be avoided. You are also in a better position to decide how long you should continue the tablets. When you find that you are getting many more nights of natural sleep than drugged sleep, then you should have little difficulty in stopping the tablets altogether, possibly keeping a few for 'emergencies'. There are many people who sleep better because they know they have a few sleeping tablets in the house. They may never use them again but the knowledge that they are there gives added security, and we have already found out how important security is to good sleep.

If you have been taking sleeping pills for many months or years and wish to stop them, what should you do?

The first thing to realize is that you are almost certain to have temporary problems when you stop or even cut down the tablets. If you are on the kind of tablet that cuts down or prevents REM sleep you will have stored up a great need for extra dreaming. As soon as you stop the tablets REM sleep will take up a much greater part of your natural sleep until you have made up all the loss. Getting back to a normal sleep pattern will take many weeks and in the meantime you will be more disturbed and restless at night and your sleep will not be so satisfying. As well as this you can have further insomnia because you are missing the comfort of your nightly pill (psychological dependence) or because your body is crying out for the tablet it has got so used to having (physical dependence). What you must not do is to mistake any of these temporary causes of insomnia for the type of insomnia you had before you ever started taking sleeping pills. Otherwise you will assume that you still need the tablets and will go on taking them indefinitely.

You are therefore unlikely to be able to stop your regular sleeping pill suddenly and get away with it without suffering some reaction. Most people find it better to reduce their pills gradually by taking a half or even a quarter of a tablet less every few nights. This can be done in your own time and may take many weeks, but as long as you keep on reducing it does not matter how long you take. All this time you will be getting rid of those accumulated tablets in your body and helping to get over any temporary withdrawal feelings. Many people find the most difficult stage is cutting out the final quarter or half tablet. By this stage you have overcome most of the difficult problems of withdrawal and it is only the psychological barrier of stopping the tablets completely that is holding you up. Some find it extremely difficult to cut down their tablets, particularly if they are barbiturates.

In this case it is often easier to gradually replace the barbiturates with a less addictive sleeping pill and then to reduce the new tablet. Your doctor will be keen to help you stop your barbiturates and can advise on the best tablets to take in their place. Although it takes a lot of determination and stamina to stop sleeping pills when you have been taking them regularly for over six months, success will more than repay the effort involved.

It does no harm for everyone concerned with sleeping pills to feel guilty about them from time to time. The drug companies who make and sell them deserve reproach for failing to detect the dangers of drugs such as thalidomide and of addiction to barbiturates, the doctors who prescribed them so readily in the past now wish they had been more cautious, and the insomniac at the end of the line often has cause to regret that he ever took a sleeping tablet. But we must keep a sense of proportion. Most of the sleeping tablets that are prescribed now are quite safe and if they are taken correctly and for as short a time as possible they are most valuable. If as much thought went into the taking of a sleeping pill as is taken with some of the other treatments for insomnia, then many of the problems would be avoided. The pill is the easy answer because it apparently needs no effort on your part. But if you take it without thought now, you will more than make up for it in thought and effort later. Above all, when you take a sleeping pill remember that it is not a cure for insomnia, it is only a temporary solution.

To come back to our comparison with taking aspirin for toothache. If you need a pain-killer several times in one day when you have toothache you are not going to ignore the causes of your pain. At the same time as' taking your aspirin you will probably arrange an appointment with your dentist to check your teeth and arrange for the right treatment for the toothache. This treatment may be filling the tooth, extracting it, or draining an abscess, or the toothache may have another medical cause. The treatment the dentist gives will be a cure if the cause is an infected tooth which needs to be removed, but the aspirin you take to relieve the pain is not. Look on the sleeping pill in the same way, as a temporary relief, but do not forget to look for the cause of your insomnia. It is not so easy as finding the cause of toothache but it is definitely worth searching for.

Some Odd Aids to Sleep

It would take a full eight hours of good sleeping time to list all the remedies for insomnia that have been recommended through the ages. Most of them are of doubtful value, but their variety and inventiveness are another way of telling us how common insomnia is and how ineffective our treatments have been in the past. It also warns that a treatment for one person may be quite useless for another, which is hardly surprising in view of the many causes of insomnia.

Food, drink and sleep have often been linked, sometimes in peculiar ways. In the seventeenth century one of the treatments for insomnia was 'the juice of lettuce mixed or boiled with Oil of Roses, and applied to the forehead and temples', which for some reason was not advised in 'those that are short-winded, have any imperfection of the lungs, or spit blood'. If you used your garden lettuce in this way your friends would think you had taken leave of your senses. Unlike many old herbal remedies this particular one has been shown to have no scientific basis. Great attention used to be paid to bowel disturbance as the source of many illnesses and insomnia took its share.

Constipation was blamed for many cases of insomnia and a good clear-out with laxatives was recommended before going to bed. But laxatives can bring their own problems and this practice is not advisable, particularly as the time of bowel action cannot be predicted.

The importance of settling the stomach before going to bed was also thought to be very important. Avoidance of all food and drink containing acids such as fruit and wines was suggested, and the taking of bland foods like milk and bread was recommended. For most people this advice is not necessary, but for those with stomach trouble such as ulcers it is worth following. One of the favorite aids to sleep is peppermint water, possibly because it settles the stomach and cuts down all those grumbling noises which can often seem to get deafening when you are trying to get to sleep.

Herbs have been used in the treatment of insomnia for many years. They persist today in hop pillows which can be bought in many stores. The principle behind herbal pillows is not really clear. The smell is fairly pleasant, if you like that sort of thing, but very strong. Your sense of smell gets tired out by strong odors and after a while the herbal pillows smell rather like ordinary ones. Perhaps helping to get your sense of smell exhausted also exhausts the rest of you and helps in getting off to sleep. I can find no record that herbal pillows and herbs in general have been tested properly in insomnia and as they have been used for centuries and continue to sell, there may be something useful in them.

One explanation for their value which most of their supporters would quickly deny is that they only work in smelly bedrooms where the smell of the herbs is needed to counteract all the other odors.

Pillows also have a folklore of their own. They can be bought in a bewildering number of shapes and sizes wedge- shaped, rounded (which keeps its shape even with your head lying on it), contoured (so it fits your head perfectly) and inflatable ones, which are often used by campers and hikers as a matter of course. A great deal of nonsense is written about the best pillows for sleeping and you would do best to rely on your own judgment. The shape of a pillow when you lie on it depends on your weight and the type of filling in the pillow. Some prefer a hard pillow, others a soft one, and many insist on having no pillows at all. Apart from people with some medical conditions in which support for the head and shoulders is often advised during sleep, there is no reason why any particular pillow should be preferred.

Electricity and magnetism have always held a fascination for insomniacs, and there are many theories about their importance in sleep. We discussed earlier the odd ideas about bed position and good sleep. The insistence that some have about placing their beds so that they sleep in a north-south or east-west line comes from magnetic principles.

Magnetic lines of force run in a north-south direction; they are lines that we cannot see and as far as we know do not influence us. However, recent work has shown that birds probably are affected by these forces and use them when migrating, so we should not be too skeptical about them affecting us in some way as well. But we know that magnetism does not change our brain waves and there is no evidence that it can influence sleep. The same superstitious belief is behind the success of sleeping-aids based on magnetism.

Magnetic pillows are among the more curious. The idea of these is that magnets inside the pillow will send impulses to the brain and help sleep by removing tension and anxiety. Of course the idea is nonsense and the pillows can only help the insomniac if he believes that they will help his sleep. You might think it is unfair of me to take away someone's touching faith in these pillows by writing this, but magnetic pillows are not cheap and belief can be achieved much less expensively. The same kind of claims are made for electro-sleep, a treatment which involves passing small pulsating electric currents from the front of the head to the back. The currents used are small and only produce slight tingling sensations.

Electro-sleep is quite different from electric shock therapy, a treatment which is used for some forms of mental illness, particularly severe depression. Before electric shock therapy is given the person has to be put to sleep by an anesthetic and there is no memory of the treatment. In electro-sleep therapy the person is fully conscious during the treatment and immediately afterwards, and there are no unpleasant after-effects. This type of treatment has been popular for many years in Eastern Europe and Russia and has created interest in the United States.

Although it has been practiced in many forms for the past century, people became much more interested in the treatment when it was shown that in many animals there is a sleep center in the brain. When the sleep center is given a direct electric current the animal goes off to sleep in a few seconds. Sleep is more complicated in man and it is not possible to pick out an area of the brain and call it the sleep center. Nevertheless, some areas of the brain are concerned with sleep much more than others and it is quite possible if a small electric current was passed directly to these areas has been given to insomniacs they do not go to sleep immediately, but it is claimed that they feel drowsy soon afterwards and then pass into a natural sleep.

This sounds impressive but the effects do not last. For example, in a recent American test, twenty out of twenty-four insomniacs had improved sleep after a course of electro-sleep treatment but two months later only eight of them were still improved. When electro-sleep has been compared with a dummy treatment (in which no electric current was given) there has been no difference between the two methods as far as relief of insomnia was concerned.

So electro-sleep has not been proved to be of any use in helping insomnia, and this is hardly surprising. When a small current is passed between two points on your head it takes the easiest route, over the surface of the scalp and not through the brain. So the sleep centre, even if it exists, does not get any direct stimulation.

'But thousands of insomniacs have improved on electro sleep, so it must be doing some good', protest the supporters of the treatment. The reason why so many sleep better after the treatment, and also why this improvement does not last, is almost certainly because it has a good 'placebo' effect. Remember when we read about sleeping pills and noticed how powerful were the effects of a dummy pill if you really believed it would help your insomnia. Now just imagine if a shiny black box with different color wires attached to it was placed by your bedside. A band with metal pads attached is fixed to your head and the wires connected to it. You are told that when a switch is turned on you will feel a tingling feeling in your scalp. This will not be painful and afterwards you will feel relaxed and sleepy. If a tiny pill has such a powerful placebo effect this treatment from the realms of science fiction is going to have a ten times greater one.

You cannot help being impressed by the magical nature of the box and wires and, sure enough, you do feel sleepy after the current is passed. But, as we know, placebo effects do not last long, so if the treatment is continued for several nights it does not impress you so much and your insomnia may return. This happens so often with electro-sleep treatment that success through suggestion must be the only explanation. Of course, if you only use the treatment occasionally it may be effective for years, but just a few nights of failure will shatter the illusion. One well-used treatment for insomnia is massage.

Eighty years ago this was one of the most respectable cures for sleeplessness. Vigorous massage was given to the stomach, thighs and legs to improve the circulation to the lower parts of the body. This was quite different from the gentle massage that is often given nowadays for relaxation, and its aim was to divert blood away from the brain. Hot compresses were placed on the stomach to encourage the circulation still more. The brain was thought to be deprived of blood by this technique and so it stopped working temporarily. In other words, you went to sleep. Although this theory of sleep has been shown to be nonsense, the fashion for massage still persists. In this electronic age you can buy automatic massagers which shake the bed and mattress from side to side as though you were sharing it with a pneumatic drill. Perhaps the idea is to give you some healthy physical exercise so you eventually go to sleep through exhaustion. The massagers also have loud whirring motors which get tedious after some time and may also help your sleep. Gentle massage sounds to be much more comfortable and you can get something very similar to it when you sleep on a water bed. Although the water bed is most often considered for medical conditions in which a long period of rest in bed is necessary, it can be a help to insomniacs. Each time you turn over the bed gently molds and caresses you so that you are always comfortable and relaxed. There are no bumps or lumps and you feel suspended in cotton wool. It is both a pleasure to sleep and lie awake in a water bed.

Contact with water in one form or another is common among sleep remedies. It may reflect the ideas of going back to the womb that are so often compared with sleep.

You will already know about the relaxing effect of a hot bath and even this has been commercially exploited. There are special bath salts sold for insomnia which are claimed to relieve tension and make you ready for sleep. But you can no more absorb bath salts through your skin and relieve tension than you can help sleep with juice of lettuce boiled with Oil of Roses, so if you buy bath salts it should be for other reasons. Hot water remedies often compete with cold water ones for sleeping. Our tough Victorian forefathers recommended a cold bath before retiring (and on getting up in the morning) and hydrotherapy was one of the most favored treatments for insomnia. Nowadays hydrotherapy is a treatment involving exercise in a warmed swimming bath and is used for many muscle and joint diseases. But in the past hydrotherapy included hot, cold, tepid and salt baths, and the application of compresses and wet packs to the head, chest, stomach and other parts of the body, and was often the main treatment for diseases such as asthma, pneumonia, scarlet fever and nervous disorders for which no other remedies were available.

The theory behind hydrotherapy for insomnia was to cool the brain down so that it did not get over-excited. An excited brain meant sleeplessness and a cold, wet pack pressed 'to the forehead cooled the brain down so that you could sleep.

This is why you see so many old drawings of sick people lying in bed with a sad relative sitting with wet cloth in hand, ready to dab at regular intervals. It is worth knowing about these old remedies, even if they are now part of history, because they show how fads and fashions can dictate treatment if there are no really good remedies available.

Acupuncture is now being considered seriously in western countries as an aid to insomnia and many other conditions. Like yoga, the theory of acupuncture is very difficult to translate into anything that makes good scientific sense, but there is excellent evidence that it works. In particular, acupuncturists appear to be able to help chronic severe pain which, as we noted before, is often the main cause of insomnia.

Acupuncture clinics are now beginning to spring up in many places and if conventional medicine has failed you then they may be worth a visit. The same can also be said of osteopaths, who are not medically qualified, but who are often skilled in removing muscle and joint pains by manipulation and similar treatments. But beware of charlatans, and try and get a recommendation from someone who has had experience of treatment. There are many people who exploit the gullible insomniac by promising sleep with worthless goods, from lucky charms to pillows which inflate and deflate, sounding like someone breathing beside you. Before you buy any gadget designed to get you to sleep, remember the warning about placebos.

The more impressive, and more expensive, the treatment, the more likely you are to have a placebo response. In other words, the treatment will always work at first and you will swear how marvelous it is, how it was worthwhile selling the car to buy it, and recommend it to all your friends. But a few weeks later it will be a different story, and your latest purchase will go to the store room where all the other instant aids to sleep have been discarded. All treatments of insomnia that work immediately and completely should be looked at with suspicion. Perhaps you should look into your mind rather than your purse and think a little more when you hear of the next 'breakthrough' in sleep devices.

If you do, you should make a saving in money as well as sleep.

How to Deal with your Insomnia

This final chapter is for insomniacs; those who have a curious interest in the subject for its own sake can give it a miss. At the beginning of the book I emphasized that to tackle insomnia properly it had to be investigated systematically. In previous chapters we have learnt about the different causes and ways of treating insomnia; in the this last one we need to bring them altogether in a master plan.

Although there are almost as many forms of insomnia as there are people suffering from it, there are some general rules we can follow in getting rid of the problem. Before describing the plan I must add that there are no guarantees attached, only a fool or a seller of sleep gadgets guarantees good sleep for all insomniacs. The plan follows six stages of investigation which are followed in order. Do not cut out any of the stages even if you are convinced they do not apply to you.

STAGE 1 - Are you a true or a false insomniac?

There is no point in going beyond this stage unless you are really suffering from insomnia and not just complaining of it. False insomnia is common and you need to ask yourself honestly whether all or part of your sleeping difficulty is an exaggeration of normal sleep habits. An independent check of your sleep by your wife or husband can often prick the bubble of your apparent insomnia. If you get off to sleep within twenty minutes of going to bed and only occasionally wake in the night, others can put your worry into perspective and show you it is quite unnecessary. For some people with active minds twenty minutes is a long time when you have nothing to do but get to sleep, and it seems more like twenty hours. Another way of checking whether you really have insomnia is to ask yourself whether you have had any of the persistent symptoms of sleep lack that were described in the third chapter. All of us have difficulty in concentrating, feel irritable, cannot remember as well as we should and have headaches occasionally, but when you have them are they usually related to your difficulty in sleeping the night before? Do you find yourself needing catnaps during the day to keep going? If you cannot relate your insomnia to these symptoms, or rarely have any of them, then it is unlikely that your insomnia is genuine.

One reason for saying you have insomnia when you really have no difficulty in sleeping is that other people give you more attention than they might otherwise. This is very difficult to admit to yourself and it might even be true without you being aware of it. But just think carefully what your life would be like if you did not have your insomnia. Would your husband or wife see less of you? Would you have less to talk about to your friends and neighbors? Would other people have to stop treating you like an invalid and more like a healthy person? If you have true insomnia these questions will all have strong negative answers, and you will probably think it ridiculous that they are being asked at all. But if the thought of losing your insomnia makes you feel uncomfortable and you are not certain about your answers to these questions, then it is quite possible that your sleeplessness is false. This does not mean there is no problem, but it is not in the insomnia territory. You may find your life so boring that it is only your regular visits to the doctor, the anxious questions about your health and sleep from your spouse, and the company of fellow 'sufferers' in the yoga class that make it interesting. And if you say you feel tired. during the day because of lack of sleep, others are more likely to do all those chores that you would like to avoid. If your insomnia is used merely to gain advantage, you can only solve it by facing up to this less pleasant part of your nature. You can change, but only if you stop deceiving yourself as well as others.

There is another kind of false insomnia which is important to recognize. Some people cannot get to sleep because they go to bed at the wrong time. Unlike the other kinds of false insomnia there is real delay in sleeping but it's quite different from that of true insomnia. If you go to bed at ten o'clock and stay awake till eleven before going off to sleep, then awake after a good night's sleep at seven in the morning, you could be in this category.

Your sleep pattern is quite normal but you are going to bed before it is necessary. We mentioned earlier that there are great differences between the hours of sleep that people need. There are similar differences in sleep rhythms. Some have a rhythm of 'early to bed, early to rise', a habit much preferred by our Puritan forefathers, who added the words 'makes a man healthy, wealthy and wise'. In fact, the late owls who do not go to bed till the early hours and wake late in the morning, are no better and no worse than the early sleepers. What you need to do is to recognize your normal rhythm, the rhythm of sleeping that you would adopt if you were left entirely to your own devices, and try and keep to it. From time to time other demands such as those of young children, different working hours and the sleep rhythm of your sleeping partner may alter your times of going to bed, but try and return to your normal rhythm as soon as possible. This does not mean that your rhythm is absolutely unchangeable, but that you should take it into account with all the other things that are necessary for good sleep.

STAGE 2 - Why are you not sleeping?

Deciding on the cause of your insomnia is often much more difficult than deciding how to treat it. Because of this you might be tempted to skip this stage altogether, but you would be ill advised to do so. Finding the cause and removing it is by far the best way of removing your insomnia, although to begin with it may be more difficult.

Although the many causes of insomnia have been discussed earlier, you may have difficulty in recognizing them as responsible for your insomnia. It is usually more difficult when your insomnia has continued for months or years and of course several causes may be involved. What you must do is to have a completely open mind about the matter. Some people like to have everything cut and dried and tend to blame their insomnia on things they can touch, see or hear. They are the insomniacs who will spend hundreds of pounds on sleep aids to cut down noise, make the bed more comfortable, keep the temperature of their bedrooms absolutely constant and so on. They think of sleep in the same way as they think of an electrical circuit. If all the connections are right the current will flow.

If you cannot sleep, they argue, there is something wrong with the mechanics of sleep. These people find it very difficult to think of emotional causes of insomnia because they cannot get to grips with worry, depression and anxiety in the same way that they can with the creaky springs of a mattress.

Others of a hypochondriacal nature will tend to put down all causes of insomnia to disturbances of physical health. They are the ones who will be certain that if they wake up in the night and feel short of breath, they have heart failure and need urgent treatment. When they get headaches because of their insomnia their minds will automatically turn to morbid thoughts about brain tumors or strokes. On the other hand, there are still others who will always find a psychological cause for every complaint, from in growing toe-nails to diabetes. There is a joke about the psychiatrist who decided to take on a patient for treatment because he was absolutely normal.

As he was the first person he had ever seen who was normal he decided there must be something badly wrong.

I have come across several examples of this kind of thinking and feel the original story must have been based on fact. Although you would like to think that you fit none of these stereotypes and are well balanced in your attitudes, it is likely that you tend towards one more than the others.

You probably have blind spots which could prevent you from seeing obvious causes for your insomnia. So even if you think you know exactly why you are having difficulty in sleeping, it is still worthwhile asking other people who know you well whether they agree with you. This applies even more if you have searched your mind and cannot find any reason for your sleep problems.

The type of sleep disturbance often helps in finding out its cause. The commonest type of insomnia is difficulty getting off to sleep and this can have dozens of causes. But waking after getting off to sleep is only found with a few conditions. Everyone wakes in the night occasionally but if you cannot get off to sleep again afterwards it becomes insomnia. If when you wake up you feel absolutely wretched, think that life is not worth living or even think of suicide, then your insomnia is almost certainly caused by a depressive illness. These are not the mild feelings of depression that everyone has from time to time, but a mental illness that needs treatment. With this type of illness self-help is not enough and you will need to see a doctor.

Similarly, if you wake up in the night with difficulty in breathing and this continues for many minutes after waking, you probably have a physical cause for your insomnia. Waking in the night with severe pain in your stomach is common with duodenal ulcers and this will also need medical advice. Sleep is natural and uninterrupted, and waking in the early hours of the morning may be a signal that something is badly amiss. If this is the nature of your sleeping difficulties you should seek professional advice sooner rather than later.

STAGE 3 - Take away the cause of your insomnia

Again this is much easier said than done. If the cause is one of the straightforward problems mentioned in the chapter on self-help there will be little difficulty in removing it, but most causes will be more complex. Early morning waking, as we have noted, will often need medical advice. It is important when you go to your doctor with a problem like this that you tell him all the relevant details. If you just say you have difficulty in sleeping without saying more you might only receive a prescription for sleeping tablets. You should not always blame the doctor for not asking you more questions. The average general practice consultation lasts only six minutes and many can have as little as two minutes. If you have early morning waking you need to stress this and also describe your symptoms, feelings and thoughts when you wake in the night. This is not a problem to be dealt with by sleeping tablets, as these will only obscure the real cause.

If you decide that you are not sleeping because your life is badly wrong and that a complete change is needed, then you will have to talk about this further with your wife or husband, friends and other relations. You may be right, and a change in job, moving house or a new relationship will bring back normal sleep again. But you may have mental illness such as depression which could have affected your judgment. This will need some treatment but not the radical changes that you mistakenly think are the only solution. If, of course, your insomnia is judged to result from shift-working with its frequent changes to your sleep rhythm, then it is quite reasonable to try and return to regular day-time (or night-time) work.

Many insomniacs will be quite certain of the cause of their difficulty in sleeping. They know it is worry and if they are asked kindly to stop worrying they are inclined to reply acidly that if they knew the answer to that their sleep problems would have disappeared long ago. It is these insomniacs who are inclined to rush off into treatment prematurely without looking for and removing the cause of their worry. In a few cases it is true that insomnia itself is the cause of the worry, but you must not take this for granted. Many people find the clues to the cause of their worrying from the thoughts that go round in their minds while they are impatiently waiting for sleep, or from analysis of their dreams. Dream analysis is a complicated subject and there is a lot of argument about the meaning of dreams.

Bearing in mind that you only remember a small proportion of your dreams and that these are distorted a great deal on waking, it is not surprising that they can be interpreted in many different ways. There used to be a fashion for sexual interpretations of dreams, coming from the work of Freud, who claimed that hidden sexual conflict was the cause of much mental illness. Dreams showed this conflict in symbol form, so apparently unimportant dream material was really a coded message from the unconscious. For example, many sharp or protruding objects such as arms, legs, noses, umbrellas, knives, spears, posts, hats, screws and cigarettes are symbols of the penis, and hollow containers such as rooms, boats, cups, mouths, shoes, boots, and glasses are symbols of the female sex organs.

Going for a walk, a ride in a bus or train, entering a room, travelling by lift, closing an umbrella and getting dressed are all symbols for sexual intercourse. You can see the many possibilities of dream interpretation from an ordinary dream of the previous day's activities from the following example (the interpretations are in brackets): 'You get up in the morning, swing your legs (penis) out of the bed and get dressed (intercourse). You go downstairs into the kitchen (intercourse) and have a boiled egg (penis) and a cup of tea (female sex organs). It is raining so you get out your umbrella (penis) and put on your boots (female sex organs). You walk down the road (intercourse) and wait at the bus stop (penis) until a bus comes. You travel by bus (intercourse) to town and go into the office (intercourse) where you have a glass (female sex organs) of water.' So now you know why you feel tired at the end of the day!

This sample of dream interpretation is a little unfair on the psychoanalyst, whose techniques are rather more subtle, but it illustrates the dangers of self-analysis of dreams. But this does not mean that you cannot assess your dreams in a more straightforward way. For example, one lady I know with persistent insomnia had a recurring nightmare of being attacked by the town hall in which her husband worked. She was sure she was taking second place to her husband's job and felt neglected and annoyed with him. These thoughts were in her mind frequently, so even if you regard dreams as a mere 'running over' of the day's events the dream could be interpreted in the same way. The content of the dream is then a reminder of your problem and suggests that something needs to be done about it, rather than a flash of insight about an unknown difficulty. So however you look at dreams, they have something to tell us about ourselves, and we should not ignore them.

Once you think you have removed the cause of your insomnia, there is an immediate check on whether you are right or not. If you sleep well again you have hit the jackpot; if you remain sleepless you will need to try again.

STAGE 4 - Is your insomnia acute or chronic?

By this stage I hope we have lost several insomniacs on the way, because their difficulty in sleeping will have been solved at its source. But I suspect most will still be reading on because they feel, rightly or wrongly, that the cause is too complicated to pick out and remove, or they know it only too well but can do nothing about it. The next stage is an easy one. Has your insomnia lasted for more or less than two weeks? If it is two weeks old or less, we can regard it as acute insomnia, if more than two weeks, it is chronic insomnia. The period of insomnia has to be continuous for more than two weeks before it deserves the chronic label, so one night of insomnia every week for a year would still be looked on as acute.

STAGE 5a - Treatment for acute insomnia

Do not bother to read this if you come under the definition of chronic insomnia, because it will probably confuse you.

The acute insomniac only has occasional difficulty in sleeping, usually at times which are predictable. So if you are in this group, you may know well in advance that you are likely to have difficulty getting off to sleep the night before a wedding in the family, a long journey, a visit from friends or relatives, a public performance of any sort such as acting or speaking, and any other event which you regard as important, no matter how trivial it may be to others. These are the occasions when you say to everyone that you must go to bed early and have a good night's sleep, but instead you lie awake for hours.

Other occasions when acute insomnia may be a major problem include extreme forms of stress; times when you have been shocked by something completely unexpected and just cannot adjust to the change. Again the cause of the insomnia is as plain as a pikestaff, but you cannot do anything to relieve it. Examples include being involved in a serious car accident, having a close member of the family being taken ill suddenly, and hearing unexpectedly that you have lost your job. These are not quite the same as the 'big occasion' insomnia, because you know it is going to take at least a few days to adjust to the change.

At these times you need to have at your disposal a way of getting off to sleep which is safe, reliable and simple. Ideally you should have used it before and realized its correct use and limitations, but of course there has to be a first time. Any of the techniques described in this book can be used. You are the one who decides which is the most valuable for you. It may be that your regular attendance at yoga classes has been well spent, and that you can turn away your mind from unpleasant thoughts and feelings when required. Or you have perfected the technique of auto-hypnosis, with or without the aid of a tape-recorder by your bedside. Or maybe the relaxation exercises that you have mastered will soothe those tense, aching muscles and allow you to sink into sleep.

Perhaps the easiest of all these methods is the taking of a sleeping pill as it involves much less effort on your part. This means that it is more often used than it should be, but if you are to take sleeping pills this is the most appropriate type of insomnia for them. The choice of pill should include the tablets such as those for sea-sickness, which are not usually thought of as sleeping pills but have similar effects. If you have never taken a sleeping tablet before and feel on occasions like these that it is absolutely necessary, then it is wiser to choose one of the sedatives which are normally used for treating anxiety. These include Valium and Librium and their fellow drugs, or alternatively a sea-sickness pill such as Avomine. There is tremendous variation between the effects of a tablet from one person to another and it is always preferable to have some idea of what previous feelings you had after taking the tablet. So if you have taken a tablet for an allergy or for motion sickness and it has made you very drowsy, you are likely to be very sensitive to the effects of most sleeping pills and should take them only in low doses. If you take a normal dose you are likely to oversleep and have severe hangover problems the next day.

There is one other warning. If you find that a sleeping pill is the only way you can cure your episodes of acute insomnia, you may keep a bottle in your medicine cabinet and only take out a tablet once or twice a year. At this rate you will take several years to get through the bottle. This may be dangerous, as some tablets deteriorate as they get older and very few will remain unchanged indefinitely. If you are getting a prescription of sleeping tablets for this purpose from your doctor it is wise to have a small number at a time. This will also remind you that they are not to be taken regularly.

The dangers of taking the tablets regularly should by now be clear to you. Try and work out a plan before you take your first tablet which decides for how many nights you will take the tablet and what dose you will take each night. For most occasions you will need to take the tablet for one night only and almost never for longer than a week, during which time you will be reducing the dose.

Once you have found your best way of treating acute insomnia, stick to it and avoid trying many others. A little self-learning can be a dangerous thing and it is always best to stay within the bounds of your own experience.

Whatever method you choose to treat your acute insomnia, go at it vigorously. You will find that if your insomnia continues and becomes chronic, it will be much more difficult to treat.

STAGE 5b - Treatment of chronic insomnia

When insomnia becomes a regular problem the original cause often pales into insignificance beside the new problems created by and continuing the sleeplessness. In treating chronic insomnia we are therefore concerned with breaking the habit of not sleeping as much as with trying to control or remove the problem that started it off. We can therefore take short cuts by giving help in sleeping while trying to solve the problem causing it. But we must always do both and not just be satisfied with sleeping well again. This advice may sound odd, for surely the whole idea of treating insomnia is to get normal sleep back again. This is true, but so many of the treatments for sleep do not give normal sleep and if you are going to use them night after night you will quickly run into problems. The most obvious example is the sleeping pill. This does not give natural sleep and if you take it regularly for more than a few weeks you are likely to have some difficulty in stopping. For many forms of mental illness it is helpful to have good sleep with the aid of tablets, but this is only one small part of the treatment and will never be given alone.

Before treating your insomnia you also need to know how much harm it is doing. There is no point in overreacting to a regular delay in sleep of one hour after going to bed. This, if it really is one hour, is genuine insomnia but is not serious. One way of dealing with it is just to accept that you have this delay in sleeping and allow for it. This often begins an important change in attitudes because it means that you no longer worry about going off to sleep. When you stop worrying, sleep is closer and may creep on you unawares. If you are having very little sleep at night and feeling wretched during the day because of shortage of sleep, then something more radical needs to be done. Let us assume that you have tried all the forms of self-help and techniques described in the earlier chapters.

You cannot find the cause of your failure to sleep and are getting to the end of your tether. Each night seems to be worse than the night before and you dread going to bed. If all these things are true you have a serious problem and almost certainly you will have other complaints such as severe pain, feelings of panic, anxiety or depression and hopelessness. The key difference between this and more straightforward insomnia is that it gets steadily worse. As we found out earlier, sleep and waking are finely balanced and it is only in physical and mental ill-health that the scales are tipped so the balancing mechanism no longer works. In this case you will have to ask for professional advice. Most people will have no qualms in going to a doctor if pain is stopping them from sleeping, or if they know they will just receive a sleeping pill. But they baulk at talking about mental troubles.

If you have them as well as insomnia, and have to go to a doctor, do not wait for him to extract the symptoms, but come out with them so he knows the full story. If you leave your six minute consultation with only a prescription for sleeping tablets you will have done him, and yourself, a disservice. You will creak along with these until another crisis forces the real problem to the surface, and by then valuable time will have been wasted.

Fortunately very few of the chronic insomniacs reading this will fall into this group, which can rightly be called ill.

Most will have a persistent sleeping problem which changes a little from week to week but which never gets really out of control. It is something that subtracts from their full enjoyment of life but does not take pleasure away altogether.

The cause may be lost in the mists of the past or may be something beyond the powers of the person to alter, his worrying personality, his hypersensitivity to noise, his tendency to turn things over and over in his mind, no matter how trivial they are. Obviously if he has gained something from the sleep remedies described earlier he will use them, but as we have found, the longer these techniques are used the less effective they tend to be. If you feel you are getting nowhere with them there are other things you can do. First try and break up your nightly routine a little. Although the pre-sleep rituals are often important in getting good sleep they have the opposite effect if you fail to get to sleep after following them. So change the time of going to bed, go out in the evening instead of staying at home, get involved in that hobby which you keep on putting off till you have more time (or more sleep).

Take a little more exercise so that you are physically tired by the time you go to bed. The amount of change is probably more important than its nature. You need to break the habit of insomnia by association, and this means removing all those things from your life that remind you of those sleepless hours.

There is an even more dramatic change you can try, particularly if you are sceptical about my repeated statements that sleep is natural and will always follow when you are sleep-deprived. One weekend, when you have nothing important to do the next day, try staying up all night. Do not go to bed, drink plenty of hot coffee or tea, and get down to some activity like working out a problem. Walk up and down every so often to keep yourself awake. Go outside and see the sun rise if it is summertime. It is marvellous to hear the dawn chorus on a fine morning-it sounds quite different when you are lying in bed cursing the birds for making so much noise.

By the time the milkman arrives you will be ready for breakfast and will probably feel quite alert. You may even marvel at your powers of concentration as you read the morning paper, and wonder whether you really need any sleep at all. But as the day goes on you will find yourself getting drowsier and noticing that you are generally less efficient. You may even be tempted to have a quick nap.

Don't. You must try and stay awake till the evening as this is essential if your next night's sleep is to be a good one. As the night draws on you feel sleepier. Take in the feeling completely, remind yourself how delightful it is to feel completely tired, relaxed and ready for bed. Sit and read for a short time in bed, look around you and see how much friendlier the bedroom seems than it did before. I promise you that when you finally turn off the light you will have a deep and satisfying sleep, provided you have not cheated and had a quick nap at some time in the previous twenty-four hours. You can use sleep-deprivation positively to get your normal sleep rhythm back, and of course the sleep you have is completely natural sleep, without any side-effects.

I have managed to get nearly to the end of this book without mentioning one of the most famous remedies for insomnia, counting sheep. I have nothing against sheep, and quite enjoy counting them in sheepdog trials, but have seldom met anyone who actually uses this traditional way of coping with insomnia. This is not to say that mental exercises are not helpful in preparing you for sleep.

To be successful they have to be utterly useless and insoluble. It is no use going to bed with one of the real problems of the day which cannot be solved, it has to be some brain-teaser that completely confuses your mind till it becomes exhausted and gives up in disgust. Then you are asleep. There are many published mental puzzles that you can try but if you are a chronic insomniac you will quickly exhaust them and will have to invent your own.

Some find repeating something. over and over in their minds is effective, others have to think in visual images, mathematical symbols, word puzzles such as anagrams, or in time riddles. Choose the type of problem that makes you most muddled and disorganized and off you go. It is as well not to put too much effort into it as this will only keep you awake. And always make sure in advance that there can be no definite solution. If you make a mistake and find the solution just before the magical point when you drop off to sleep, you will be completely awake again, and find you have answered the wrong problem.

STAGE 6 - Making the most of your insomnia

If you reach this stage you will feel that you have failed in your quest for sound sleep. You have not, but let us assume for the moment that you have. Accept that you are going to have insomnia for the rest of your days and there is no point in getting het up about it. You will know from reading this book that you are not going to get really seriously short of sleep, because your mind and body will not allow you to go that far. So insomnia is an inconvenience but is not fatal, and you are going to make the most of it.

One of the things that annoys you most when you are trying to get to sleep and failing miserably is that you are wasting time. As you know only too well, the time spent while waiting to go to sleep seems to pass extremely slowly. It passes slowly because you are bored. You have tried auto-hypnosis, yoga, relaxation, meditation, listening to the radio in or under your pillow, counting sheep and doing innumerable puzzles in your mind, but you have done it all before and any novelty they had has long since disappeared. Why waste all this valuable time?

Instead of going to bed and trying to get to sleep, go to bed assuming you are going to be awake half the night. It is like a long train journey; you will need to take something with you to help pass the time. If you are a slave to work you might take some papers to bed and work on them, or if you wish to enjoy yourself more take a good book, not a boring one, to bed with you and really get stuck into it.

Try doing crosswords, finishing off your knitting, filling in your tax return, writing letters, planning your next holiday. It does not matter what, provided you can do it while sitting in bed. As you work or enjoy yourself think positively about all the advantages you have over the other poor duffers all around who are sleeping. You are stealing a march on them; by getting things done now you are giving yourself extra free time in the day. They are wasting their time sleeping while you are using it constructively. As soon as you get bored change over to something else that holds your interest more. You will be surprised how quickly time goes by. From time to time you may feel a little tired or you may find the light in the bedroom too bright.

Why not turn it off, you can think just as well in the dark. Think about what you have been reading or doing, and remind yourself that concentrating late at night and taking in new knowledge is much more effective than when you do it by daylight. You are taking in a great deal more. But if you start getting bored again turn on the light and do something else. Have a bit to eat if you are hungry, turn on the radio and listen to some fascinating programmes, knowing that no one else in the street is lucky enough to be in your position.

Listen to the sounds of the night outside. Learn to identify the owls by their characteristic hoots, and the lark as it tells you happily that daybreak has come. If it is silent, let the silence sweep over you, reminding yourself that so few others in this busy world can be as lucky. From time to time you may think about sleep from force of habit. After all, it is what you usually thought about before you realized the positive aspects of insomnia. Don't let your mind dwell on it for too long, because it will start to become boring and time will go more slowly again. If sleep comes it will do so at its own discretion and not at your bidding; and if it does you may realize with annoyance the next morning that it came just at the critical point of the novel you had been reading, or just as you were knitting the last row of the jumper.

You were interrupted by sleep, not rescued. It takes a little time to turn the tables on insomnia and use him to your advantage. But once you have sampled his delights you need no longer be afraid of him. If he comes in the night you should look on him as a welcome visitor as he gives you a chance to catch up on all those things you have been meaning to do but have been unable to find the time. He is no longer the bogeyman that has you cowering in your bed praying for oblivion, but a friend whom you know well, although he visits less often than he used to. And if you are not frightened of his knock, you will sleep all the more soundly when he decides not to call.